This Giving Birth

This Giving Birth:
Pregnancy and Childbirth
in American Women's Writing

edited by

Julie Tharp
and
Susan MacCallum-Whitcomb

Bowling Green State University Popular Press
Bowling Green, OH 43403

Library of Congress Cataloging-in-Publication Data

This giving birth: pregnancy and childbirth in American women's writing /
edited by Julie Tharp and Susan MacCallum-Whitcomb.
     p.   cm.
    ISBN 0-87972-807-8 (cloth) -- ISBN 0-87972-808-6 (pbk.)
     1. American literature--Women authors--History and criticism.
    2. Women and literature--United States--History. 3. Mother and child in
literature. 4. Childbirth in literature. 5. Motherhood in literature.
6. Pregnancy in literature. I. Tharp, Julie Ann. II. MacCallum-
Whitcomb, Susan.
PS147.T55 1999
810.9'3520431--dc21

                                              99-051805

Cover design by Dumm Art

To Ana and Ian, Duncan and Sophie

who made us mothers

CONTENTS

INTRODUCTION

Now that the baby boom generation has come of age in America, mothers are suddenly back in *Vogue*—and in *Time, The New Yorker,* and *The Wall Street Journal* too. Indeed, mothers are suddenly everywhere, and their influence is everywhere felt. Pollsters and policy-makers court them; manufacturers cater to them; and corporations work to accommodate them. Marketers adjust to meet their demands and desires, while medical practitioners keep pace by emphasizing prenatal education and offering non-traditional birthing options.

Ever since a pregnant Demi Moore exploded the beauty myth by posing nude for a magazine cover and Madonna cast off her boy-toy image to sing the praises of maternity, popular culture has also begun to embrace dear old mom. Books are written about her, and "after years of cinematic attention to unmarried women, working girls and fatally attracted predators," movies are again treating her as "an interesting character—a star—in her own right" (Merkin 104).

Even in the spiritual realm, mothers are enjoying a resurgence. Mary, the original Madonna, is hailed with more enthusiasm than ever, and assorted maternal goddesses have become the focus for new-age seekers. But motherhood and, in particular, issues related to pregnancy and child-bearing, have not always been so widely accepted.

In 1980, a mere two decades ago, Sharon Olds performed an "exceptional act" when she published a poem about her experience with pregnancy and childbirth. Admittedly the physical process she discusses, as miraculous as it may seem to the individuals involved, is commonplace. Women, after all, have been giving birth for thousands of years. Moreover, the poem in question was, even then, only one contribution to a rapidly growing corpus of work. What made Olds' "The Language of the Brag" remarkable was that it detailed the corporeal reality of pregnancy and childbirth, shying away from no bodily function, and it did so in a way that was unsentimental, unembarrassed, and, most importantly, wholly unapologetic.

Given that the occurrences described are so central to the "lives of one half of humanity" (Kizer, "*Pro Femina*" 44) and until recently have been silenced or privatized, Olds' poem represents a watershed in that it examines the ways in which childbirth has shaped both a woman's identity and her imagination. Through "The Language of the Brag," Sharon

1

Olds redefines the birthing experience, giving voice to feelings otherwise devalued in patriarchal societies; she forcefully confirms that pregnancy and childbirth are legitimate subjects for literature; and, in doing so, she issues a challenge to a culture that has routinely used the language of birth for everyone and everything except the actual event.

The poem opens with Olds recounting her adolescent search for "some epic use" for her "excellent body." It concludes with her mature realization that the maternal role is, indeed, an heroic one. Thus, in the final stanza, Olds can celebrate the fact that she has "done what you wanted to do, Walt Whitman,/Allen Ginsberg:"

> . . . I have done this exceptional thing,
> I and the other women, this exceptional
> act with the exceptional heroic body,
> this giving birth, this glistening verb,
> and I am putting my proud American boast
> right here with the others. (45)

The knives she throws with her "exceptionally strong and accurate arms," particularly those directed at Whitman, hit their mark. In "Song of Myself," this nineteenth-century poet who has been praised as a great egalitarian wrote of the "exclamations of women taken suddenly who hurry home and give birth to babes." To his credit, Whitman asked, "What living and buried speech is always vibrating here, what howls restrain'd by decorum" (30). But rather than encouraging others to listen for those muffled exclamations buried under patriarchal debris, or indeed stopping to listen for them himself, Whitman decided to speak for the "Maternal as well as paternal" (36).

Envisioning himself as the only possible transmitter of "long dumb voices" (41), Whitman sang the "song of procreation" (69). Convinced that he was pregnant with truth, he "chant[ed] the chant of dilation" (39) and gave birth without "the obstetric forceps of the surgeon" (46). Then, having nursed his offspring with "seminal milk" (77), he pronounced himself to be the "most venerable mother" (132). In short, Whitman did everything save letting living, breathing mothers speak for themselves. In the process, he stole the language of birth, and in this he was not alone.

Karen Haas-Howland provides her own attempt to reclaim that language in our opening essay "The Circular Journey of Poetry and Children." In this meditation on the role of pregnancy and childbirth in her writing process, Haas-Howland situates herself within a community of women writers, past and present, who have also wrestled with the apparently conflicting demands of motherhood and writing. What she discovers, both through the writers she quotes and her own work, is that in fact these roles are complementary, bringing new insights to both endeavours. The creative form of the essay suggests that being a "motherpoet" may require a shift away from traditional, linear writing and, instead, a move toward more circular, bodied forms of writing. It may give rise to other unique hungers as well.

Our second essay offers the reader some historical background in which to situate writing like Haas-Howland's and that of the authors she cites. In "Bringing Forth Life From Body to Text: The Reclamation of Childbirth in Women's Literature," Michele Lise Tarter chronicles some of the major religious, scientific, and cultural discourses of childbirth which historically pre-empted their narratives. Tarter makes abundantly clear that men have been simultaneously appropriating maternal metaphors and denigrating the authentic maternal voice for centuries. Quoting extensively from primary sources, Tarter reveals the strategies employed to rob women of their power and of the deafening quiet which was created as a result.

Susan MacCallum-Whitcomb examines this phenomenon by focussing on the ways in which it has operated specifically within the context of American literature. In "Claiming Our Birth-Write: The Poetry of American Mothers," MacCallum-Whitcomb argues that American poetry long upheld a distinctly male model of experience which viewed motherhood as an artistic liability. Beginning with the country's first poet, Anne Bradstreet, she recounts how the maternal voice was suppressed by the "Great Men" of American letters. But she also demonstrates how literary mothers in the twentieth century struggled to reinvest maternal discourse with an authority lost since pagan times.

That their struggle has been successful is now beyond doubt. One need only look to new anthologies on the literature of motherhood for proof that birthing comprises both a thread running through much of women's literature and, more recently, a central focus for women's writing. Laura Chester provided one of the first such anthologies with her *Cradle and All: Women Writers on Pregnancy and Birth* (1989); four others followed soon after: *In the Gold of the Flesh: Poems of Birth and Motherhood* (1990) edited by Rosemary Palmeira, *The Book of Birth Poetry* (1995) edited by Charlotte Otten, *MotherSongs: Poems For, By and About Mothers* (1995) edited by Gilbert, Gubar and O'Hehir, and *Mothers: Twenty Stories of Contemporary Motherhood* (1996) edited by Katrina Kenison and Kathleen Hirsch.

These collections of creative writing are complemented by a number of critical studies which view the issue of motherhood from different perspectives. Tess Cosslett's book, *Women Writing Childbirth:*

Modern Discourses of Motherhood (1994), Kathryn Allen Rabuzzi's *Mother and Child: Transformations Through Childbirth* (1994), and Robbie Pfeufer Kahn's *Bearing Meaning: The Language of Birth* (1996) are a few of the recent works which simultaneously foreground the importance of such anthologies and complicate our readings of them.

We can, conceivably, locate the origins of this re-naissance in the *fin de siecle,* feminist classic which is the subject of Gail Lippincott's paper, "Thirty-Nine Weeks: Pregnancy Imagery in Kate Chopin's *The Awakening.*" Lippincott examines how the novelist privileges the language of birth, employing a double-voiced discourse which allows her to structure her work according to the rhythms of pregnancy. Of course, Chopin, like her character Edna Pontellier, paid a high price for her subversive behaviour: the novel was considered so scandalous that her career was ruined. Nonetheless, she did serve as a midwife of sorts, for her efforts enabled later writers to bring their own creative work to term.

By the 1920s, for instance, Mina Loy had the confidence to state outright that "Nature endowed the Complete Woman with a faculty for expressing herself through all her functions" (270). Even the more conservative Amy Lowell could maintain that while the ability of any woman to combine motherhood and literature still seemed "miraculous" (459), it was, at least, possible. She believed that women were potentially "double-bearing,/With matrices in body and in brain" (459), and in her lifetime this belief was beginning to be put into practice.

Still, obstacles remained as Debra Beilke demonstrates in "Southern Conceptions: Feminist Procreation in Julia Peterkin's *Scarlet Sister Mary* and Frances Newman's *Hard-Boiled Virgin.*" Dealing with two little known writers of the 1920s, she argues that Peterkin and Newman had to struggle with the ways in which motherhood both shaped and distorted women's identities in the post-suffrage era. In exploring this anxiety, Beilke notes that class and race particularly influence the female protagonists in the social and psychological choices they feel are available to them.

It is, of course, no coincidence that the strengthening of the maternal voice coincided with the battle for women's rights and, more specifically, reproductive choice. Just as it is easier to celebrate pregnancy when no social stigma is attached to it, and to celebrate child-rearing when economic hardship is not a pressing concern, it is easier to celebrate motherhood in general when you have the freedom to decide whether or not you'll have children in the first place. Despite the advances made in subsequent generations, these questions have never been entirely resolved. Women writers must still contend with the admonishment of their peers, both the men who believe that "Women artists fail/Because they have babies" (McDonald 189) and the women who believe that "motherhood is the sinister invention/of patriarchy" (Ostriker 46).

Consequently, some of the writers best qualified to use the "glistening verb[s]" gained from maternal experience continue on in silence (Olds 45). This is particularly true for those American women who remain bound by the patriarchal assumptions of their culture. In this collection, for instance, the voices of Asian-American and Latina mothers are not heard. Many other women, however, have consciously chosen to speak in "The Language of the Brag."

Especially in the years since World War Two, American women have, in increasing numbers, become "double-bearing" (Lowell 459). The post-war period, when women were expected to make the transition from Rosie the Riveter to June Cleaver, was crucial because it forced many mothers to turn to creative writing as the only available means of self-expression. These literary pioneers began to speak of motherhood and the "problem that had no name" long before Betty Friedan coined the term in 1963 (Friedan 11).

A large proportion of today's literary mothers were, in turn, influenced by the women's movement of the 1970s and early 1980s. Although their works are highly individualistic, all of these writers have given pride of place to the maternal subject. They have asserted the power of the authentic maternal voice, and, in doing so, reminded us all of the political nature of personal experience.

Nowhere is the overlapping of the personal and political more apparent than in the writing of African-American women. Andrea O'Reilly delineates Toni Morrison's "theory of mothering," emphasizing the importance of the motherline in the formation of the African-American woman's identity. She begins by contrasting characters who have experienced the benefits of traditional black motherhood with those who suffer a disconnection from it, and concludes, as Morrison herself does, with an affirmation of maternity as an integral component in the empowerment of black women.

Brenda Daly's consideration of incest and female characters' bearing of their fathers' babies complicates this vision. Both of the novels Daly examines, *Push* by Sapphire and *Thereafter Johnnie* by Carolivia Herron, portray characters who resist and even reshape institutional powers, of family, of language, of actual agencies, in order to create a world that will honor them, that will allow them to claim their babies. Daly is interested in the power of these books to challenge the seeming neutrality of language, particularly as it relates to the body and taboo subject matter.

Julie Tharp's paper, "'Into the Birth House' with Louise Erdrich," focuses on another kind of empowerment, this time within the context of the Native American community. Erdrich, she argues, celebrates the human need for inter-connection by bringing not only biological families together but also joining people over time, space, and profound personal differences in a complex web woven from the stories of the characters' origins. Tharp shows that while Erdrich refutes "any primitivist fantasy of Indian women's childbirth," she presents birth stories as sources of regeneration, crucial for any sense of connection with the creation.

In "'Some Epic Use for My Excellent Body:' Redefining Childbirth as Heroic in *Beloved* and 'The Language of the Brag,'" Ellen Argyros looks back both to Toni Morrison and to Sharon Olds, the poet who gave this anthology its title. According to Argyros, these two writers ask us to reconsider the criteria for heroism and, in so doing, reexamine the birth acts of women as heroic. Underlying the challenge, Argyros says, are two specific objectives: the desire to valorize the experience of ordinary women and the desire to make a place for the writers of maternity literature in the established canon.

Finally, we offer another creative essay, this time by poet and literary critic Kimberly Blaeser who reflects on the role pregnancy and childbirth have played in her development as a "poetmother." While similar to Haas-Howland's essay in its personal style, Blaeser examines both practical changes in her life, like the time she has for writing, and more esoteric ones, like the shift in her linguistic register and the structures of maternal writing. Blaeser's dual writing careers provide a balanced look at the demands placed upon women in her position, women asked to be not just "double-bearing," but in some ways triple-bearing. Learning to bear those many burdens creatively may be the greatest contribution mothers can make today.

Taken together, the articles which follow record the difficulties women have faced as they worked to transform themselves from objects into maternal subjects, as they fought to fill the silence with their own "vibrating" songs (Whitman 30). Both the quality and the quantity of material dealt with in these pages demonstrates the extent of their success. Nevertheless, literature is grounded in reciprocity, so the battle cannot truly be won until readers fulfil their part of the creative contract by altering their own perceptions of maternity.

Of course, some will continue to resist making this paradigmatic shift—and with good reason. As Alicia Ostriker asks in "Propaganda Poem":

    . . . who can bear the joy that hurts nobody
the dazzling circuit of contact without dominance
that by the way makes you less vulnerable
to cancer and who knows what other diseases
of the body
because who can bear a thing that makes you happy
and rolls the world a little way
        on forward
           toward its destiny

"Who," Ostriker goes on to ask,

    . . . can tolerate the power of a woman
close to a child, riding our tides
into the sand dunes of the public spaces. (44)

We hope that the answer soon will be "everyone."

Works Cited

Bradstreet, Anne. *The Complete Works of Anne Bradstreet.* Eds. Joseph R. McElrath, Jr., and Allan P. Robb. Boston: Twayne, 1981.

Chester, Laura, ed. *Cradle and All: Women Writers on Pregnancy and Birth.* Boston: Faber and Faber, 1989.

Cosslett, Tess. *Women Writing Childbirth: Modern Discourses of Motherhood.* Manchester, England: Manchester UP, 1994.

Friedan, Betty. *The Feminine Mystique.* New York: Dell, 1963.

Gilbert, Sandra, Susan Gubar, and Diana O'Hehir, eds. *MotherSongs: Poems For, By and About Mothers.* New York: Norton, 1995.

Kahn, Robbie Pfeufer. *Bearing Meaning: The Language of Birth.* Champaign, IL: U of Illinois P, 1996.

Kenison, Katrina, and Kathleen Hirsch, eds. *Mothers: Twenty Stories of Contemporary Motherhood.* New York: North Point P, 1996.

Kizer, Carolyn. "Pro Femina." *Mermaids in the Basement.* Port Townsend, Washington: Copper Canyon P, 1963. 41-51.

Lowell, Amy. "The Sisters." *The Complete Poetical Works of Amy Lowell.* Boston: Houghton Mifflin, 1955. 459-61.

Loy, Mina. *The Last Lunar Baedeker.* Ed. Roger L. Conover. Highlands NC: Jargon, 1982.

MacDonald, Cynthia. "Instruction from Bly." *No More Masks!: An Anthology of Twentieth-Century American Women Poets.* Ed. Florence Howe. New York: Harper Perennial, 1993. 188-90.

Merkin, Daphne. "Rethinking Mom." *The New Yorker* 1998. 104-05.

Olds, Sharon. *Satan Says*. Pittsburgh: U of Pittsburgh P, 1980.

Ostriker, Alicia. "Propaganda Poem: Maybe for Some Young Mamas." *The Mother/Child Papers*. Santa Monica: Momentum, 1980. 42-47.

Otten, Charlotte, ed. *The Book of Birth Poetry*. New York: Bantam, 1995.

Palmeira, Rosemary, ed. *In the Gold of the Flesh: Poems of Birth and Motherhood*. London: Women's P, 1990.

Rabuzzi, Kathryn Allen. *Mother and Child: Transformations Through Childbirth*. Bloomington: Indiana UP, 1994.

Whitman, Walt. *Complete Poetry and Selected Prose*. Ed. James E. Miller, Jr. Boston: Houghton Mifflin, 1959.

1

THE CIRCULAR JOURNEY OF POETRY AND CHILDREN

Karen Haas-Howland

Our poems often circle us, years before we consider them. They are inside us in a similar way to how our grandmothers carry us in their bodies the last five months of their pregnancy. Our egg rests secretly within her daughter who dreams in *utero*. In the fourth month of fetal development, a female is given all of the eggs she'll ever have, showing the vast creativity and fertility that cycles throughout generations. From grandmother to mother to daughter, we circle, spinning wonderful lines from inside our bodies as we hang from the highest branch, suspended above everything we've ever desired.

* * *

> Your day approaches.
> The pears fatten like little buddhas.
> > Sylvia Plath, "The Manor Garden"

Stretching between the apple and pear trees in my back yard, the iambic pentameter of a hammock holds my body. Here. There. Near. Far. You. Me. Watching the delicious curve of pear flesh swell with light, I feel my belly and forget what I am exactly. In this sweet moment I could be a pear. Held in that metaphor, I merge, I draw my shape over and over invisibly in the air, connecting the pears with my finger, as my intricate shape shifts in the west wind, as the boundaries of things sweet, disappear. My body, my baby, my poetry: it's all fruit waiting for reality to ripen. I wait. I sway. We widen when we write.

I see them everywhere! Pregnant women. Life bulges generously and I can't stop it. I see hills surfacing in the landscape, melons piled next to the eggplant at the farmer's market. Even my poems swell.

I'm obsessed with round letters, anything with an O. Obese, oblong, oblivion, ocean, open, ooze, oracle, oak, odor, oncoming, omnivorous, opiate, oppressive, orbit, organism, orgasm, osmosis, other, offspring, outpour, out of print, out of one's mind, oval, ovum, overjoyed, overburden, overreact, oversleep, overcast, overwhelm. When will the nine overblown months be over?

For three weeks I can't read because of the fierce nausea that resembles motion sickness. I can't even ride a mile in the car without hurling, so I wait on the couch as the DNA inside me spins faster and faster. Without moving I travel to the land of mother. Hormones have hijacked the muse. There needs to be a new Olympic category for expectant mothers who are nauseated. We train with saltines, eating thousands. We do deep knee bends. We grow huge. We hurl. We prepare for the great event, the one that will challenge us unlike any other.

I cannot write for weeks as I listen to this strange genetic language repeat itself. I try to crack the code of who she will be. I drink chamomile tea and see the word "mom" suspiciously wedged within. Everything reminds me of what I am becoming. I see forms and words and shapes in a different way. I see with a mother's eyes the molecular level of poetry.

A baby develops, divides, multiplies at a rate exceedingly fast. I grow slower. As I sleep, poems develop, divide, and multiply. Words take root in cells, tremble within marrow, and gestate imagination. On one level, I never feel this fattening, but my blood responds intuitively, nourishing this new life.

As the poem recognizes my voice under the vivid water of the unconscious, does it somersault when I say good morning? At what point can the poem hear, feel pain, or retract when it hears my words? When a poem reaches a certain stage of maturation, is it suddenly aware of me? In Linda Hogan's poem "Shelter" she writes:

> Downstairs, my daughter sleeps.
> There is only a thin, closed eyelid
> between her and all the rest.
> A dream
> I am to her.
> I am just large and dark,
> the woman who feeds her.

Why couldn't the words become aware of the women who care for their forms, protect their integrity, and nurture them with a mother's energy?

* * *

The shape of a cave, the bud, the chrysalis, the shell, what new form we seek in this darkness . . . what we seek here, warm and covered with water, we sweat in this effort. . . . This cave, the shape to which each returns.

Susan Griffin, *Woman and Nature*

When I enter the cave of labor, I want to be comfortable with the dark, dripping horror. I want to dip my hand in my own blood and draw on the wall the totem of a mother bear. I don't want to be pressed against a sterile field, flat on my back, feet in stirrups, spine and spirit numbed. I want to squat like an Aztec goddess spitting out obscenities a doctor would never tolerate. Who ever heard of a woman having a creative experience under fluorescent lights, surrounded by busy faces and metal forceps?

I'll have the baby at home in my place of power, where I write, work, cook, and make love. I want to birth her with my own sweat, effort, focus, as the strongest muscle in the human body, the uterus, releases her mystery. I want to trust my own rhythms and birth her in our own time. I will listen to my rhythm for it will never again feel this primal. This visceral understanding of how rhythm really works within poetry won't come easy. Breath. Wait. Allow. Push. Separate. Release.

I will be Demeter, determined, going great distances to find her daughter. Unlike her, I will go underground where words ferment. I will take one between my teeth, crushing it as I say "Mother." I will become the mother bear on the cave wall as the moment of birth consumes me, as you Persephone return from the dark, red loam between my legs. I will feel a rhythm older than words, as I become rhythm, a moan, a moon, remembering the woman I am within this Logos, this Loba, this Love, this effervescence called daughter that leaves the cave. A new word will be born wild and howling.

* * *

I have lain down and sweated and shaken. . .
this giving birth, this glistening verb.

Sharon Olds, "The Language of the Brag"

There is this fear mothers have of our water breaking in the most awkward place, like along the communion rail. There is this fear writers have of inspiration leaking out at the most inopportune time. Suddenly, I'm in the grocery store considering cantaloupes and it happens, the poem comes glistening out as I grip the cart, hoping no one noticed. Secretly, I want them to notice and exclaim, "My god, she's about to have a poem. Clear the way," as they carry me out. As it turned out, my amniotic water proved much more discreet than my poetry, giving way in the privacy of my home.

* * *

> . . . may the taste of salt
> recall to us the great depths about us.
>> Denise Levertov, "The Depths"

There were depths I reached during labor where divers, astronauts, and nouns never go. Plunging underneath everything I'd ever known informs my body of a rhythm which erupted when volcanoes first gave lava to the sea as fire leaped into our spine, a heat creating us out of salt and spark.

During labor, inner and outer landscapes join in the salt of it all, in the sweat of everything. As I pushed for the third hour, exhaustion took me down. Lost in the dark stillness I felt the roots of the cottonwood tree behind our house. I began drawing strength from the roots as I reconnected to a deeper source. I felt my flesh turning into a powerful tree. This went beyond metaphor. Reality actually shifted as I drew on the earth from where I'd come. Her head finally crossed the threshold in my turbulent song of muscle, vulva, and blood. I was comforted when I realized that my daughter was drawing her breath from the red tree-shaped placenta she grappled beneath. For nine months, all she'd known was the sustenance of this tree inside me which had planted itself from pure instinct.

Later, because our life depends on looking at both afterbirths, poetic and placental, we lay the red fragments out on the table to see if any part of the poem is missing, amazed at the tender complexity of poem-making. The process of discovering the parts that still might remain in the mother is vital. If the smallest piece is missing, a hemorrhage occurs and the poem and I lose our lifeblood.

Now that the poem has arrived humble and entirely dependent upon me, I'm captivated by something I cannot name. Grateful, proud, and entirely spent, I lay back and instinctually bring the poem to my breast, falling asleep as words softly feed next to my heart.

* * *

> The calm-milk giver who
> knows sleep, knows growth, the sex of fire and grass,

and the black snake with gold bones.
Muriel Rukeyser, "Night Feeding"

It is two a.m. Your hunger is awake. My milk is awake. There is this music of us in the darkness. We both drink this thick moment. Words melt away as we merge. I cannot find words in this darkness so I hum. I blanket you with a song that seems to come from within, but it could belong to someone else. My mouth doesn't move. Your mouth moves. A word sparks as light flashes on the ceiling with the passing of a car. I hear you. I hear me. Neither is defined in this labyrinth of thirst. We breathe and the room seems to inflate with a dream. The room is suddenly round. The room is gone. I touch my breast. I am Silbury hill, your ancient nourishment. Your curious soul is a lamb who will not leave this warm, rising curve. The calm spaces between words were never empty, they were womb, music, the vivid curve of fire. Denise Levertov's "In the black of desire we rock and grunt, grunt and shine" echoes somewhere.

* * *

Before Chloe was born I'd ruminate the late hours away wondering how having a child would affect my writing. I knew it would be more necessary than ever to write, and I fantasized about how the process would metamorphosis. When my child cries in the middle of the night, will it be reminiscent of how poems woke me up demanding my attention at that raw, honest hour? What are the specific similarities between the birth process and the poem-making process? Do they touch upon a common mysterious shore? Will birth feel like a poem written with blood and muscle? Will I walk the floor holding poetry and a child close to my breast in the lavender shades of night, everything drenched in motion and shadow, her edge meeting mine? Will I disappear into the beat, as I step with effort to the spondaic rhythm between window and rocker? Will the rhythm itself mother me, as my body cries with fatigue?

When she finally falls asleep, will I put my mouth by her mouth, smelling the delicate aroma that tells me of a world made only of milk? Yes. Will I draw close to the poem, smelling for the same authentic aroma? Yes. Will I get pulled into a whirlwind of words, of her, of work, of diapers, of small spoons, of applesauce? Yes. Will I fall only to find myself redefined in this garden of demands? Definitely.

Months later I forget these rational thoughts and run naked to my bedroom. Hiding behind the door, I try to recognize myself in the mirror. My stomach once rose like a moon. Now I grieve as it gives way to a concave, crescent shape. Soon, I will become completely new as I disappear into this domestic sky. If I look long enough, I remember that this is just one cycle. I will reappear, rising in full form.

Saffron Goddess

She rises when light enters like an egg
    breaking across the surface of her house.
These early moments are sacrament
    the warm rushing water washing
        her journey into the kitchen
  simple mantras like cinnamon
    pulse within, without
she starts to boil water
    stares into the heat
recognizing the cauldron
    she remembers dreams
as oatmeal moistens
    against the music of grain and spoon.
The woman has been to this edge many times before
  with basil, thyme, cumin,
    cardamom, coriander
mother, daughter
    tender, death, surrender
salt, question, thirst,
    the alchemy of family.
Hands dance thanking their source
  cupped in wonder
    drinking hazelnut coffee
breathing, breaking,
    round, honey whole wheat bread
her body, pure and ready
    the baby wakes.
She touches her breast
    let there be milk!

* * *

To be a parent—an experience shattering, ridiculous, earthbound. . . . I want to fly. . . . instead, I sink roots. With ferocity and purpose and a tenacity that resembles joy.

Louise Erdrich, Blue Jay's Dance

Today I feel amphibious. I am a woman who wants to sleep. I am a writer who wants to jump poem to poem. I am a poet. I am a parent. One minute I'm breathing through the gills of letters as I swim the white expanse of the page. The next I'm running towards my crying child, both of our lungs expanding, expressing the pain that contracts us, as we fight not to feel small.

Being connected by the air of parenting and the water of writing, I am an amphibian. I am hidden away in the swamp of these first weeks like a deep-throated bullfrog whose voice needs to be heard from the dark forgotten bog. My breathing comes more quickly. Gasp. Go. Universe. Verse. Running between round words and the baby's apple-cheeks. Gulping air as if it were disappearing. Losing myself ecstatically in the poems and the moments with Chloe. Surrendering to the inspiration of both. I forget to breathe and realize this is how things shine when they first begin. Native American thought believes things begin in the middle, so maybe things always shine, maybe Chloe has always been, maybe I've always been made of words.

Gladiola Light

I wasn't prepared for my face to fall full petal apart
        after my screams   you cracked
        the moon open   smelling autumn   I saw you
        fall from me   your face breaking   bud
        from me   deep rememberings
        subtle loam   three hundred thousand tears
        before eve

                there was this beautiful woman
                        now a baby   warm within my arm
        wide with gladiola light   skin sings
        eyes speak   fir trees
        lids   tremble heavy
        fingers curl   like fire
        our mouths   howl little ooo's
        the milk   blossoms.

The poem came to me before Chloe was born. They say "write what you know" and there I was, a woman who had never experienced birth, writing about breaking full petal apart, and filling with milk like nectar by the second. In rare poetic moments, we transcend time and see into our past and our futures. Taken out of ourselves beyond the usual boundaries, we see ourselves.

The poem came to me in one piece as if it were whispered in my ear. After it finished itself, the name Chloe buzzed in my head like a bee whose legs are full of pollen. I followed that bee to its source, despite the fact that I had grad school to finish. I gave birth to Chloe on February first, almost two years to the day after I first birthed the poem.

* * *

> . . . the sea grass
> flew like a woman's hair in labor.
> Anne Sexton, "The Sea Corpse"

I now only allow myself one luxurious ritual before sitting down to write. Necessity has pared down my options. She could wake up at any second, so I must leap to my desk like a bobcat. Forget breathing deep, reading Sandra Cisneros, or lighting a candle. Now I do the one thing that I must: I brush my hair. Tipping my head upside down, taking my Aveda paddle-brush and stroking my long brown hair with Cleopatra-like pleasure, I purr. I untangle strands of dreams and redistribute their oil. I begin to gleam. I ignite as sparks fly from bristles and the radiator hisses with dry, heat oracles. I imagine my brain is being massaged and I stimulate memory, I ask things of my blood and finally there is the familiar tingle. I have reached all the way down to the roots, the corpuscles, the ecstasy. I begin writing, trying to keep the tingle.

I have learned the art of writing through interruptions. My desk is in the kitchen between jars of fettuccine and the sink. I'm accessible to the morning light, the fragrance of soup, and her curiosity. The interruptions have become sources of inspiration. Their strange timing congeals a unique combination, I never could've dreamed up without my daughter's ooo's and ahhh's. She notices a slant of light that becomes essential to the end of my poem. She says "apple" repeatedly and suddenly there is a tree in my poem. She touches my elbow and suddenly the poem bends a certain way. She edits my poems, with her feet no less, kicking my pen as it hawk-circles, crossing out a part that disappears like prey consumed for survival. Spontaneity, laughter, interruptions shatter the trance I used to covet. Instead I'm left with daughter-altered brainwaves from sleep-deprivation and too much joy.

* * *

> If a woman is inconstant,
> good, I am faithful to

ebb and flow. . . .
There is no savor
more sweet, more salt
than to be glad to be
what, woman. . . .
                    Denise Levertov, "Stepping Westward"

For centuries, fairy tales have talked of children so sweet they had to be eaten. Anne Sexton continued that thread in her poem to her daughter Linda, "Oh, little girl,/my stringbean,/how do you grow?/You grow this way./You are too many to eat." Thirty years go by and Chana Block writes in her poem "Eating Babies": "nibble earlobes, dip my tongue in the salt fold of shoulder and throat." Any new mother or obsessed poet knows the irresistible urge to blow on a baby's belly. Their delicious nature is so fresh with a beauty that must be taken in with the fingertips, palm, mouth, tasting babies as they taste us.

What if I could be that intimate with my poems, reveling in a line as if it were a skinfold, realizing the wonder of its breath, its incarnation on the page? My poem couldn't help but thrive, grow intelligent, and at last become independent of me. Like Sylvia Plath, in her poem "Child," I would pause before my poem as if it were a waiting child and say, "Your clear eye is the one absolutely beautiful thing./I want to fill it with color and ducks/The zoo of the new." The motherpoet learns to infuse her poem with a curious, four-pawed, salmon-eating power, nourishing her deepest self.

* * *

Hunger knows we have not yet reached
the black and raging depths of anything
                    Linda Hogan, "Hunger"

As a motherpoet, my hunger yearns to taste other salt-covered worlds. There are dark paths I have traveled and have yet to travel, not from ambition but from insatiability. I am pulled by unseen lines of poems that spiral relentlessly. I am comforted in circles of womanness through the return of Chloe. I am the motherpoet, reborn, and ready to give birth to more forms strange, salty, and familiar.

Flesh Passages
The passage establishes its mud and emotion
over bone, under muscle, into cell

pulsing fluid, blood-beautiful music,
adagio,
lines of skin as song
accelerando, lips open
what is ocean
what is shore
what is child
what is poetry
all life is
vivacissimo
as one
viscous cell ebbs
from heaven, from honey, from legs
that pollinate layers of this flesh passage.

Works Cited

Block, Chana. "Eating Babies." *The Past Keeps Changing*. New York: Sheep Meadow P, 1992.

Erdrich, Louise. *The Blue Jay's Dance*. New York: HarperCollins, 1995.

Griffin, Susan. *Woman and Nature: The Roaring Inside Her*. New York: Harper and Row, 1978.

Hogan, Linda. *The Book of Medicines*. Minneapolis: Coffee House P, 1993.

Howland, Karen. "Saffron Goddess," "Gladiola Light," "Flesh Passages." Unpublished.

Levertov, Denise. "The Depths." *Jacob's Ladder*. New York: New Directions, 1961.

——. "Stepping Westward." *The Sorrow Dance*. New York: New Directions, 1963.

Olds, Sharon. "The Language of the Brag." *Satan Says*. Pittsburgh UP, 1980.

Plath, Sylvia. "Child." *The Collected Poems of Sylvia Plath*. Ed. Ted Hughes. New York: Harper and Row, 1981.

——. "Manor Garden." *The Collected Poems of Sylvia Plath*. Ed. Ted Hughes. New York: Harper and Row, 1981. 125.

Rukeyser, Muriel. "Night Feeding." *Collected Poems*. New York: McGraw-Hill, 1978.

Sexton, Anne. *The Complete Poems*. Boston: Houghton Mifflin, 1981.

2

BRINGING FORTH LIFE FROM BODY TO TEXT:
THE RECLAMATION OF CHILDBIRTH IN WOMEN'S LITERATURE

Michele Lise Tarter

High upon an ancient Irish church wall, there stands a woman figure who looks poignantly down at all who pass by her as she, with powerful hands, grasps the sides of her vagina and holds wide open her womb to the living world. Worshipped for her powers of parturition—defined originally as the act of "bringing forth"—, Sheela-na-gig, a pre-Christian goddess, has survived centuries of male church elders' destruction of pagan worship in the Celtic world. A testament to the long-suppressed celebration of the divine feminine, she serves as a meticulous emblem for contemporary women in their reclamation of childbirth in both living experience and written word.

As a visual image carved on the front of the temple, Sheela-na-gig embodies ages of oral narratives that could never be told by women, due to patriarchy's historical erasure and/or control of the subject of childbirth in literary discourse, ultimately reflecting the social guards placed upon women's bodies, women's sexuality, women's procreative power, and women's voices. Yet, with her emphatic gesture sculpted centuries ago, she beckons women, even today, to give birth to their power as they bring forth life from body to text.[1]

In a recent wave of literary production, numerous writers have adhered to this call and contributed to the growing corpus of women's literature which aims to resurrect and recover the discourse of childbirth that has been appropriated by men for hundreds of years. Playwright Ntozake Shange, to name one example of many, praises her female body as the source and inspiration of her (pro)created text: "as a woman & a poet/i've decided to wear my ovaries on my sleeve/raise my poems on milk/& count my days by the flow of my mensis" (17). In a similar way, poet Sharon Olds, in her poem "The Language of the Brag," describes both the birth of her child and her poem as "this giving birth, this glistening verb" in a "language of blood" (44-45). Honoring the mystery of double creation, Shange and Olds inscribe the power granted only to women in the act of childbirth and writing, procreation and creation.

While this essay cannot possibly recount the hundreds of stories which are being retrieved and being born anew, it will chronologically historicize various religious, scientific, and cultural discourses of childbirth which have pre-empted women's narratives for centuries, and then, in light of Sheela-na-gig, celebrate the empowerment of many different women—including poets, playwrights, literary critics, scientists, anthropologists, historians, religious scholars, doctors, midwives, and mothers—as they reclaim this sacred discourse while approaching the threshold to the next millennium.

Looking at the historical reasons behind women's silenced voices and censored texts, French feminist Hélène Cixous asserts: "For if there's one thing that's been repressed, here's just the place to find it: in the taboo of the pregnant woman" (261). We might trace such a taboo back to the Judeo-Christian creation myth of Genesis: as punishment for disobediently eating from the Tree of Knowledge and thus abetting in the fall of humankind, Eve is told by a castigating God that she and all women will suffer for her sin through the curse of painful childbirth.

Western culture's traditional Aristotelian dualism, in turn, separated the sexes by associating men with the soul, reason, and the mind, and women, quite pejoratively, with the body and birthing. As a constant reminder of the fall from paradise and grace, women, set in such a binary frame, were meant to represent carnal desire and suffering to humanity. In the ensuing battle between flesh and spirit, then, men were to loathe the female body as the site of disobedience, sinfulness, decay, and mortality. While perceiving those of the female sex as potential temptresses like their foremother Eve, early church leaders ultimately focused on women's contaminating and base corporeality, as John Chrysostom so aptly illustrates in his tract, *To the Fallen Monk Theodore:*

The whole of her bodily beauty is nothing less than phlegm, blood, bile, rheum, and the fluid of digested food . . . If you consider what is stored up behind those lovely eyes, the angle of the nose, the mouth and cheeks you will agree that the well-proportioned body is merely a whitened sepulchre. (qtd. in Warner 58)

Indeed, St. Augustine declared, a woman had no more soul than a goose, and Judeo-Christian theology instilled in its followers a deep fear and distrust of female sexuality, fecundity, and power.

Biblical laws pertaining to childbearing women elucidate the connections made between parturition and pollution. As Leviticus 12:1-5 cites:

The Lord said to Moses, "Say to the people of Israel, If a woman conceives, and bears a male child, then she shall be unclean seven days; as at the time of her menstruation, she shall be unclean. And on the eighth day the flesh of his fore-skin shall be circumcised. Then she shall continue for thirty-three days in the blood of her purifying; she shall not touch any hallowed thing, nor come into the sanctuary, until the days of her purifying are completed. But if she bears a female child, then she shall continue in the blood of her purifying for sixty-six days."

Women were constructed as unclean by the patriarchal church after giving birth, and were doubly so if they gave birth to a female child.

While taboos, in turn, have been placed around women's experiences and narratives of birth, men have historically usurped the metaphor of rebirth to describe conversion into religious institutions, ever expanding their own authority in a hierarchy of God. That is, teaching women to fear and detest their bodies, many male elders throughout history have simultaneously positioned themselves as purveyors of the figurative "new birth." As one model among many, the prolific Puritan minister and writer Cotton Mather declared to his congregation:

Ministers are your Mothers too . . . Have they not Travailed in Birth for you, that a Christ may be seen formed in you? Are not their Lips the Breasts thro' which the sincere Milk of the Word has pass'd unto you, for your Nourishment? (22-23)

In her study of *Mother with Child: Transformations through Childbirth,* Kathryn Allen Rabuzzi asks her readers, "have you ever seen a nonprehistoric Western Madonna *giving birth*?" (xi). We see images of the Madonna breastfeeding often, and yet how often have we witnessed the symbol of sacred birth with a Madonna figure—one, for example, as so graphically emblematized as goddess Sheela-na-gig on the temple wall? Certainly none of the major world religions has focused on this fecundative act. When adopted by men, the experience of birth no longer symbolizes women's power, mystery, eroticism, or creation, and the message is quite clear: an asexual Madonna is the only "conception" of woman that is celebrated in the Judeo-Christian religion.

Throughout the Middle Ages, women mystics responded to this ideology in several striking ways, ultimately experiencing and writing "birth" through their somatic spirituality and a celebration of the body of Jesus. Although at first these "Daughters of Eve" were told that, as inheritors of their mother's guilt, they must deny their corporeality or femaleness in order to be saved, women of the later Middle Ages espoused an empowering and creative interpretation which linked female flesh to the humanized Christ. Writing as virgins and brides of Christ, they ascribed importance to *humanitas christi,* a theology which revered Christ's physicality. With no human father, they posited, Christ was "enfleshed with flesh from a woman; his own flesh did womanly things: it bled, it bled food [often portrayed as lactation] and it gave birth to new life" (Bynum 185). Myriad women recorded experiences of mystical pregnancy, miraculous lactation, and they represented events in Christ's life in terms of women's childbirth experiences; Margaret of Oingt, for instance, living in the thirteenth century, portrayed Jesus' suffering on the cross as birth pangs (176).[2] Consequently, these visionaries found an authoritative way to inscribe women's corporeal experiences as union with God.

Beyond the parameters of the church, however, it was difficult for women to withstand the harsh, misogynistic beliefs which pervaded society at large. Thousands of midwives and healers living in villages throughout medieval Europe were ultimately targeted by the church in a war against women's control of healing and birthgiving. When the Inquisition began, village midwives were at first included in this radically changing social milieu, granted permission by the church fathers to bless infants who died at birth. Nevertheless, the practice of this ritual, in addition to many other remedies concerning fertility, pregnancy, and childbirth, became far too threatening for the hierarchy of the men of God: the women's work overlapped dangerously with the priests' job as healer—and midwife—of bodies and souls.

In 1482, Dominican friars Heinrich Kramer and James Sprenger issued *The Malleus Maleficarum,* or *The Witches' Hammer,* a manual to be used for the hunting, discovery, and torturing of "witches." Accompanied by Pope Innocent VIII's Papal Bull, endorsing the treatise with the highest church authority, this lawbook was translated into half a dozen languages and was distributed to every judge and magistrate throughout Europe for the next three hundred years. In this text, which deliberates on the evil nature of women while concomitantly revealing men's horrific fear of female sexuality, the terms "woman" and "witch" are used interchangeably. An excerpt reads:

[That a woman] is more carnal than a man is clear from her many carnal abominations. And it should be noted that there was a defect in the formation of the first woman, since she was formed from a bent rib, that is, a rib of the breast, which is bent as it were in a contrary direction to a man. And since through this defect she is an imperfect animal, she always deceives . . . All witchcraft comes from carnal lust, which is in women insatiable. (44-47)

It is the midwives who are portrayed as those "who surpass all others in wickedness" (41). Readers are warned that these women attempt to alleviate labor pains, thus contradicting God's intended curse on womankind; they seize children at birth and offer them up to Satan; they obstruct conception in women; perform abortions; induce inordinate passion in men; and, most interestingly, they collect penises, as many as twenty to thirty at a time, and store them in a bird's nest, where the organs reportedly eat oats and corn.

The Malleus Maleficarum inspired a wave of violence directed primarily against women and female sexuality for the next three centuries, codifying the use of elaborate instruments of torture which were designed to mutilate female genitalia. The Pear, for example, was routinely forced into a victim's vagina by her inquisitors and then screwed open, causing irreparable damage to the cervix; a Breast Ripper was used during the "first degree" of interrogation to extract confessions regarding her heretical and sexual sins. These confessions, originally conceived by Kramer and Sprenger in *The Malleus Maleficarum* and then suggested to victims during torture, became a parody of motherhood itself, as women were forced to agree to having sex with Satan and suckling his familiars with their witches' teats. While mutilation of women's breasts and genitalia was common throughout this historical period, there was a tacit understanding among torturers that male victims' "members" would not be hurt, further revealing the prevalent and quite savage ferocity launched against women's procreative bodies.

Witch hunts became a thriving business, with public burnings serving as a spectacle for mass entertainment, for the symbolic purging of evil (read: female sexuality) in society, and for the reinforcement of political control by the church and state. Ultimately, the fear of women's healing power, of women's procreative mysteries, and of female sexuality itself was literally branded into humankind's consciousness with the thousands of public, ritualized burnings enacted in the town squares throughout Europe.[3]

In their study of *Witches, Midwives, and Nurses,* Barbara Ehrenreich and Deirdre English document the male encroachment upon women's healing practices, usurping and then legalizing their rights and privileges as educated men to treat parturitional women. With a newly defined university structure, women healers were forcibly excluded from any formal medical education and were systematically portrayed as charlatans who were not to be trusted; eventually, they were condemned to death as punishment for practicing their "illegal" midwifery and healing work.

A large corpus of scientific literature ensued in the seventeenth century in which men interpreted the physiology of women's bodies and the mechanics of procreation. Primarily upholding the theory of the second-century philosopher Galen, physicians and scientists hypothesized about the homologous nature of men and women's reproductive organs, emphasizing that women were simply "men turned outside in," with ovaries resembling testes, the vagina and cervix resembling an inverted penis, and so forth (Laqueur 2). This theory highlighted that men were more perfect anatomically than women because of their excess of heat which allowed their genitalia to exist outside of the body, women's remaining imperfect and hidden within. Despite this construction of male superiority, Galenic theory insisted that both male and female seeds were required for conception and insisted that women must derive pleasure from intercourse, believing that they ejaculated ova (the necessary seed) through orgasm.

Reflecting traditional dualism which persisted in medical theory, most scientists and philosophers believed that the male seed provided the spirit, while the female seed provided the matter for the conceived fetus. In 1651, however, the English physician William Harvey rejected the belief that men were responsible for the spirit of the child. Noting that "amongst Animals, some Females do procreate of themselves without a Male . . . but the Male never begetteth any thing without a Female," he privileged women and their uteruses as the origin of conception and life (170-75).

Jane Sharp, who was the first British midwife to write a manual for women on pregnancy and childbirth, published her book in 1671, titled *The Midwives Book, or the Whole Art of Midwifery Discovered, Directing Childbearing Women How to Behave Themselves in Their Conception, Breeding, Bearing, and Nursing of Children.* Sharp's widely circulated text, last reprinted in 1728, empowers women and their parturient bodies. In her chapter, "Of the Generation or Privy Parts of Women," she writes, "We women have no more cause to be angry, or be ashamed of what Nature hath given us than men have, we cannot be without ours no more than they can want theirs" (33). Looking at the homologous nature of women's and men's vessels preparing the seed for conception, she promulgates equality in this generative act—"As in men, so in women"—but then takes it one step further by highlighting the intricacy and advanced preparation of women's seed: "But women's Vessels have far more windings and turnings, hither and thither, out and in, than men's have, that the matter they bring may be better prepared" (54-55).

Later in the manual, Sharp notes the numerous ways in which women participate in the creation of life, listing the three requisites for forming a child: "1. Fruitful seed from both sexes wherein the soul rests with its forming faculty; 2. The mother's blood to nourish it; 3. A good constitution of the matrix to work it to perfection" (123). She then elaborates on the agentic capacity of the matrix in conception, describing how it contracts and "embraces" the mixed seeds,

being greedy to perfect this work, that by succession of time she stirs up the formative faculty which lieth hid in the seed and brings it into act, which was before but in possibility . . . it is not all the art of man that setting the womb aside can form a living child. (93)[4]

Sharp consequently empowers women by accentuating their inimitable role in the act of conception.

While Sharp holds much authority as a woman addressing other women, she finds it important to incorporate both scientific and folkloric ideas about pregnancy in her manual. How fascinating it is to read her "Signs that a woman is conceived with Child, and whether it be a Son or a Daughter." In addition to listing how a pregnant woman's breasts may swell, her appetite may be lost, and her menses will stop, the midwife relays that pregnant women may also "hath a preternatural desire to something not fit to eat nor drink, as some women with child have longed to bite off a piece of their Husbands Buttocks!" (103).

It can be said, indeed, that culture writes birth, and oftentimes culture writes "misconceptions," as well. Consider one early American historical period to elucidate this phenomenon. In seventeenth-century New England, where Calvinist Puritans felt deep hostility toward the body as the site of original sin and innate depravity, women suffered severely for being made the trope of body and nature in the traditional Christian bifurcation. Edward Taylor, representative of his community's state of somatophobia, referred to himself, for example, as "a dirt ball . . . a dung-hill, a dot of dung, a varnished pot of putrid excrements . . . guts, garbage, and rottenness" (qtd. in Koehler 18). In this seventeenth-century culture, sexual intercourse was perceived as quite a tense, even violent wrestling match between the male and female seeds. The woman was instructed to be passive during intercourse so that her husband's seed would master her own, win the match, and thus produce a male child— the best of all things possible. If the woman conceived and gave birth to a female, the townspeople might even consider her husband effeminate.

English obstetrical guides written by men and circulating in this early American community presented numerous advantages to bearing a male child: the woman, it was written, would be rewarded with a fair complexion, red nipples, and white milk during nursing; her delivery, moreover, would be much easier, according to the English obstetrical expert Thomas Raynalde. In the "unfortunate" event of conceiving a girl, the mother would allegedly be punished for aggressiveness during intercourse by having a pale, heavy complexion, black nipples, and watery, bluish milk. Even at birth, the midwives were instructed to cut a female infant's umbilical cord much shorter than a boy's, for they believed it would make the child modest and her genitalia narrower—both features considered more acceptable to her future husband.[5]

At the birth of her child, a parturient woman would be surrounded by women only, as men were forbidden to be anywhere near such a "contaminated" site as a birthing room (Rich 129). These "gossips"—a word which the *Oxford English Dictionary* cites from the seventeenth century as meaning women friends invited to be present at a birth— would take part in rituals with the woman to aid her in the stages of labor and delivery: a special lying-in room was designated, candles would be lit, and all women present would drink from a caudle, which was a special drink made for the duration of travail.[6]

Nonetheless, if the mother gave birth to a malformed child, the magistrates and elders beyond the boundary of the birthing room would inevitably label her creation a "monstrous birth," indelibly linking it to the woman's deviant behavior and spiritual decay. In fact, they believed that such offspring were often the result of sexual intercourse taking place during a woman's menses, perceived as the filthiest of all times in her reproductive cycle.[7] In looking at this particular cultural interpretation of pregnancy and childbirth, which persisted well into the eighteenth century, we must ask ourselves, *Do not such interpretations say more about a culture and its male interpreters than they do about the experience of childbirth among women at this time?*

Scientific narratives describing women's physiological stages in reproduction changed dramatically in the early nineteenth century with the discovery of spontaneous ovulation occurring in some mammals, irregardless of intercourse or orgasm. Comparing women to dogs under this study, theorists no longer upheld the old anatomy of sexual homologies, but rather replaced it with a biology of difference. From this determination onward, it has been argued, women were reduced to the organ which distinguished them most from men—the ovary (Laqueur 29). Menstruation was thereby characterized as "failed production" in a female reproductive economy, while women at this stage of their cycle were even compared to dogs in heat. A popular, old saying, quoted as late as 1985 in the *Review of Medical Physiology,* was, "Menstruation is the uterus crying for lack of a baby" (Ganong 63). It is interesting at this point to consider Gerda Lerner's hypothesis in *The Creation of Patriarchy* that the origins of domination occurred with men's desire to own and control women's reproductive agency, rather than with the formation of private property. In this light, all focus turned to the commodification of women and the production of children in patriarchy (8).

One might wonder how much Western culture has evolved in the twentieth century, in terms of understanding and writing about women and childbearing. In her important study of *The Woman in the Body: A Cultural Analysis of Reproduction,* Emily Martin reviews the current medical metaphors used to describe the female cycles of menstruation and menopause, with women often being portrayed as machines in contemporary medical literature. Focusing on college textbooks from 1980-1985, Martin thoroughly, quite convincingly illustrates how the language of reproductive biology is inundated with cultural stereotypes. In descriptions where conception does not occur, for example, the textbook reader is told that a series of breakdowns occurs in the female body which eventually lead to menstruation. The terminology used includes negative words such as "degenerate," "lack," "weakened," "deteriorate," "denuding," "debris," and "slough," terms all connoting failed production on the part of women. And yet, when spermatogenesis is described, positive words such as "remarkable," "amazing," and "sheer magnitude" are used to detail the process. Despite the position of these textbook editors, Martin shrewdly points out that only about one of every one hundred billion sperm ever actually "succeed" in fertilizing an egg; moreover, she notes, a large part of ejaculate is made up of sloughed cellular material, but the textbooks never include these equally important details in their scientific anecdotes (48-51). In other recent interpretations which evidence cultural stereotyping, sperm are portrayed in a plethora of performing roles: courting the egg like a suitor, struggling against a hostile uterus like a hero, lying in wait for the ovum like a hunter with prey, and being drawn by a powerful magnet as a seduced and helpless man. There, too, are quite bellicose accounts of "kamikaze sperm" acting in "Sperm Wars" (Beldecos et al. 61-76).

Most people living in "advanced" technological cultures now accept what is called a "value-free" model of childbirth: that is, a sperm penetrates the outer rim of an egg and successfully fertilizes it. Yet, what if we were to revision this model without any androcentric bias and perceive an egg choosing one sperm from many and allowing it to enter? Anthropologist Robbie Davis-Floyd explains:

You can clearly see the egg reach out with a tentacle and draw the sperm into the inner area. Then the egg penetrates the top of the head of the sperm and blows it up. Then it explodes, and its genetic material is distributed throughout the egg. Thus, the two merge into one, but the egg's role is active, agentic. (qtd. in Rabuzzi 2)

While most textbook accounts historically juxtapose the activity of the sperm with the contrasted passivity of the egg, recent revisionist studies such as Shatten and Shatten's "The Energetic Egg" acclaim the mutually active partnership of the sperm and egg in the process of fertilization (Beldecos et al. 61-76). Shifting our cultural perceptions of this widely accepted "value-free" model of childbirth could have profound consequences for women. As an agent rather than a passive victim, that is, a woman can reclaim her body and her metaphors.

Yet, how many of us continue to accept scientific metaphors of female reproduction as natural? Martin and other scholars reviewing this history and corpus of literature urge women to resist medical imagery and health practices that misrepresent and oppress them. Often treating parturient women as machines, the medical industry has fragmented women and ignored many psychological dimensions to giving birth. During labor, a woman is often told or signalled that she is not in control; even the position she is generally placed in—lying flat on her back with feet in stirrups—does not consider gravity and the instinctual motions of her body to abet delivery. When a woman opts to undergo natural childbirth, for instance, choosing to rely on the powers and even ecstasies of her own body, she is often ridiculed by domineering physicians. "Do you want to have your baby in an asparagus patch?" one doctor responded as this issue was being discussed at a public meeting on obstetric neonatology, implying a "primitive" quality often ascribed to this form of delivery (qtd. in Kahn 172).

Interestingly, many obstetricians use the term "birth from below" when referring negatively to a mother giving birth by the power of her body. In opposition to this, they have coined the term "birth from above" when referring to cesarean-section births, connoting the mastery and authority doctors assume in this medical performance (Kahn 147). Routinely scheduling cesarean-section births in this decade, doctors commonly overlook the psychological, emotional, and physical suffering women experience after undergoing this surgery. Martin's interviews with many such women relay stories of disappointment, emptiness, a sense of separation of the body from the self, a sense of violation, and a loss of control. In one of these interviews, Laura Cromwell recounts how she was advised to have a second cesarean-section birth but refused to do so, based on the pain she endured from her first one. Surprised by her resistance, a male resident attending her birth nonchalantly asked her, "Why didn't you want to have another cesarean? They cut you below, they cut you above, what's the difference?" (qtd. in Martin 65).

Clearly, women must reclaim their bodies and their stories, for millions have suffered from the scientific models of implied failure, the dualistic strategies of waste and decay, and the utter fragmentation of their bodies split off from their souls. In her study of *Bearing Meaning: The Language of Birth,* Robbie Pfeufer Kahn acknowledges the levels of ecstasy many women encounter during birth, as evidenced in photographs taken during their later phases of labor at Michael Odent's hospital in Pithiviers, France. This facility's focus is strictly on the energy and power of the mother's body as she gives birth; she is allowed to move and act according to her needs, and she generally squats to deliver the infant, working with gravity and with the employed midwives in the final stages of labor. In the close-ups of these photographs, Kahn explains, the women's faces are quite similar to those of women experiencing orgasm (84, note 84).[8] In effect, while midwifery is still outlawed in many states in America and expectant mothers are hardly told of the ecstatic dimensions of childbirth, hospitals like Odent's offer women a chance to recover the mystery of this powerful act.

The erotic dimension of pregnant women's experiences is treated as nearly a taboo subject in our culture today, originating in the traditional virgin/whore split of Judeo-Christian religious ideology. Perhaps nothing brings this to light more poignantly than a tragedy which occurred after Demi Moore posed as a nude pregnant woman on the cover of *Vanity Fair* in 1991. Writing a commentary on this event, Jimmy Breslin first responds to Moore's public pose and then offers the following sketch of a pregnant prostitute in its contrast:

On the other side of the world, the charred body of a woman almost at the end of her ninth month of pregnancy was found in an empty lot . . . in Brooklyn early in the morning of Saturday, July 13. The woman was an Hispanic in her late 20's, and she had been set afire while on her back and with her arms outstretched. The fire had burned much of the skin off her stomach, and the baby she had been carrying could be seen inside. (qtd. in Rabuzzi 116)

In presenting these two images, Rabuzzi insightfully writes that our culture's ambivalent—or repressive—attitudes toward eroticism, pregnancy, and motherhood lead some people to act out violently toward women. However, it does not so easily begin and end with prostitutes on the street; an American Medical Association report, she notes, recently stated that "the rate of domestic violence against pregnant women is . . .one of every six" (68), revealing the widespread and close-to-home occurrences of rage still being acted out on women's procreative bodies.

In seeking to restore the power and language of birth, many women have turned to a woman-centered theology which resurrects the history and metaphors of sacred fecundity, as represented in the figures of goddesses like Sheela-na-gig. In pre-Christian societies, over twenty-five thousand years ago, archaeological evidence reveals that fertility deities were worshipped and that birth was granted tremendous respect and prestige. Christine Downing's study of *The Goddess* illustrates how religion itself might have originated with the spiritual matrix of the maternal body, later made manifest in the vegetal goddesses.[9] Art historian Pamela Berger has documented research which shows that Mother-goddess statuettes, "sculpted as if giving birth," were placed in grain bins in neolithic Anatolia, rooted in the faith of women's power to bring forth life to the earth (6-7). And, archaeologist Marija Gimbutas' study, *The Language of the Goddess,* traces worship of the divine feminine in Old Europe to around 35,000 B.C., concentrating on the symbols and images of the great goddess which people actually inscribed on their bodies; she bases her findings on a transdisciplinary approach incorporating comparative mythology, archaeology, and folklore.

Feminist scholars of Christianity have also found ways of incorporating the goddess and reuniting the body and spirit in their religious exegesis. Mircea Eliade, a religious historian, explains that Christianity began in Judea under Roman rule during the last century B.C., a time when there were many religious practices influencing this nascent religion. The cult of Isis, she indicates, worshipped one of the most popular goddesses of the Greco-Roman world at this time. Promising salvation, Isis was often represented nursing her son on her lap, an image which Elide posits early Christianity incorporated into its iconography.[10]

Retrieving these buried images is one way of granting women a dynamic reconnection to spiritual origins and meanings, rooted in and through the body of creation. One of many manifestations of such a spirit-filled life is found with Una Kroll and her choice to live "A Womb-Centred Life":

I want to share with others the experience of learning to live and pray with the mind and heart centred in the womb. When I speak about having a womb I am using the word to describe more than an organ . . . [it is] an amalgam of elements in a woman's life which give her the ability to describe herself as a woman even if she is either born without a uterus or loses it during her lifetime . . . it is my belief that her perspective which is womb-centred is also God-centred because she is created in God's image. (93-94)

In her study of *Women Writing Childbirth: Modern Discourses of Motherhood,* Tess Cosslett summarizes that, historically, we have been given two official discourses of childbirth: one by the medical experts and the other by natural childbirth experts. Cosslett adds a third, unofficial story, the "old wives' tale," passed down in oral tradition by women such as the midwives and witches (3-4). She implores women to recover maternal subjectivity by inscribing their own experiences of childbirth into cultural literary production. Only in the last fifty years have women begun to break the relative silence about childbirth in literature. Specifically, during the second wave of feminism, around 1965, there began an explosion of women's writing about the continuum of maternal experiences, including conception, pregnancy, labor, childbirth, postpartum experience, and motherhood itself (Friedman 86).

Rejecting medical discourse which has historically fragmented women, Emily Martin has interviewed women to ask them how they would like to give birth, what imagery and metaphors come to them in remembering the experience, and what technology would best suit them, as women. She presents the plethora of metaphors women have developed in response to being asked such sensitive and subjective questions: labor is described as a river and a ripening fruit; it is compared to the acts of surfing, making love, running a marathon, and skiing down a mountain; and contractions are catalogued as "rushes" or bursts of energy (157-58). In Barbara Katz Rothman's study, *In Labor: Women and Power in the Birthplace,* labor is even described as "moving a grand piano across the room: that hard, but that satisfying, to feel it moving along" (20). Martin suggests, finally, that women can confront, challenge, and replace the medical models which desacralize birth and fragment women's bodies by creating new birth imagery, founded in their own experience, their own language, their own stories of creation.

Breaking the silence, breaking the taboo, women are now taking part in the transgressive and subversive activity of writing the female body. Hélène Cixous declares:

Woman must write her self: must write about women and bring women to writing, from which they have been driven away as violently as from their bodies . . . Woman must put herself into the text—as into the world and into history— by her own movement. (243)

French feminism, in effect, celebrates the discourse of childbirth, of women writing the body, in an "impregnable language that will wreck partitions, classes, and rhetorics, regulations and codes" (Cixous 256). While these scholars are exploring the nature, function, and power of the maternal body and mind, as women writing in milky white ink, there are anti-essentialist feminists who oppose this line of thinking, declaring it biologically deterministic and regressive to feminism by its resorting back to dualistic strategies. Yet, in *Of Woman Born,* Adrienne Rich urges us not to dismiss the body in our conception of women's knowledge and language. She expands:

In arguing that we have by no means yet explored or understood our biological grounding, the miracle and paradox of the female body and its spiritual and political meanings, I am really asking whether women cannot begin, at last, to *think through the body,* to connect what has been so cruelly disorganized . . . There is for the first time today a possibility of converting our physicality into both knowledge and power. (290)

Perhaps French feminism is not an essentialist trap if we begin to revision the role of the body in the production of subjectivity and consider the significant connection between embodiment and writing.

Ahistorical in concept, however, the theory of *l'ecriture feminine* ignores differences among women across cultures and through time, and it doesn't account for the myriad birthing stories; for, as we know, no two are ever quite the same. Scholar Carol Bigwood speaks of the dangers feminists face, however, as their fear and distrust of essentialism virtually silence many women's voices and stories:

When one looks at the long list of feminists accused of different kinds of essentialism, one fears that the recent move to purge the last vestiges of essentialism from feminism might be in danger of turning into a kind of gender theory inquisition whereby certain kinds of feminist theories are silenced as heretical. (17)

We cannot bear another inquisition in this history of women's bodies and women's voices. In the debate between essentialism and cultural determinism, potentially translated as a debate between body and culture, Paula Cooey asks if we aren't replicating an old and quite patriarchal model yet again. Rather, she warns, feminists need to reject such dualistic thinking and focus on the "inseparability of nature and culture" through women's lived experience (28-30). Women's stories of childbirth are a vital, lifegiving channel for building such bridges.

Feminist political theorist Mary O'Brien writes that history begins with humans being born, and it is to women that this procreant act has been given. She asserts, "To the question: Where does feminist theory start? I answer: Within the process of human reproduction" (8). Indeed, as Robin Morgan extols in *The Anatomy of Freedom,* "we are back to beginning where each of us began—in the female human body, the 'first home' of every human being" (42). Reclaiming home in the twenty-first century, women will inevitably reshape, redefine, and reinscribe motherhood. Some theorists suggest turning to D. W. Winnicott's object relations theory to oppose dualistic thinking and focus on the mother-infant relationship. Others encourage us to turn to childbirth rituals in non-Western cultures where this experience is treated as a sacred event. And still others urge us to embrace women's particularity, their "carnal knowing" distinct and separate from men, with the power of birth in all of its erotic and mysterious glory.[11] Texts borne out of such positionality will challenge cultural scripts of passivity and fragmentation, and offer future generations of women the opportunity and the gift of wholeness, wisdom, and new life.

Looking at the corpus of North American woman-centered birth narratives evolving in the past few decades, scholars such as the ones in this anthology are reading these texts in terms of female subjectivity and the process of negotiating identity. Many questions arise from looking through this revisionist and feminist lens: as women authors write the process of birth, be it in a fictional character or in a nonfictional account, how do they define or create the self as their bodies are changing and becoming two? Do they defy cultural prescriptions, as they concomitantly recover maternal subjectivity? How do these women negotiate their identities amidst prevailing ideologies of motherhood, and how much of their writing of childbirth is influenced by the ideas and values of men? Do these stories hold the power to provoke readers to effect change for women, and how do they include/exclude those women who cannot or who consciously choose not to bear children? Finally, are these writers negotiating with the official stories of childbirth, or is it possible for them to write in their own voices, as women, in what Sharon Olds names a "language of milk," a "language of blood"?

Tess Cosslett writes that birth "disrupts our categories," as one becomes two and one's center becomes "diffuse, multiple, fractured" (118). She continues: "Whether figured as a death or a heroic rebirth, childbirth is, however, always a turning-point, a narrative crisis that destroys, confirms or creates a woman's sense of identity" (154). Parturition, the act of bringing forth, carries over to literary creation, and we as readers behold women writing themselves into history, reinventing themselves as mothers, and literally saving themselves through the generative act of telling their own stories. Approaching the next millennium, we might ask how this body of literature will evolve as women face the challenges of future scientific recreations of birthing through surrogacy, genetic experiments, and perhaps even cloning. "This giving birth, this glistening verb" is inscribed in its own language of blood, written over and over again by women reclaiming their power—fecund, pregnant, and full. In honoring this process, we may only dream of how woman-centered narratives and inscriptions of childbirth will benefit society at large, while Sheela-na-gig continues to look upon us with all of the power of her fecund body resting in her hands.

Notes

1. Feminist historians, literary scholars, and anthropologists are currently gathering a great deal of information regarding pre-Christian goddess worship. Sheela-na-gig is one of many female deities discussed in this critical research of reclamation. See Barbara Walker, *The Woman's Dictionary of Symbols and Sacred Objects* (New York: HarperCollins, 1988); Merlin Stone, *When God Was a Woman* (New York: Barnes & Noble, 1976); James J. Preston, ed., *Mother Worship* (Chapel Hill: U of North Carolina P, 1982); and Cynthia Eller, *Living in the Lap of the Goddess* (New York: Crossroad, 1993).

2. For a detailed and very insightful reading of medieval women's mystical experiences and texts, see Caroline Walker Bynum's *Fragmentation and Redemption: Essays on Gender and the Human Body* (New York: Zone Books, 1991) and Elizabeth Robertson, "The Rule of the Body: The Female Spirituality of the Ancrene Wisse," in her *Early English Devotional Prose and the Female Audience* (Knoxville: U of Tennessee P, 1990).

3. Numerous scholars analyze the cultural construction of witchcraft during what feminist scholars call "the burning times," or the Inquisition. See, for example, Anne Llewellyn Barstow, *Witchcraze: A New History of the European Witch Hunts* (San Francisco: Pandora/HarperCollins, 1994); Diane Purkiss, *The Witch in History* (London: Routledge, 1996); Erica Jong, *Witches* (New York: Harry Abrams, 1981); Barbara Ehrenreich and Deirdre English, *Witches, Midwives, and Nurses: A History of Women Healers* (Old Westbury, NY: The Feminist Press, 1973); Mary Douglas, ed., *Witchcraft: Confessions and Accusations* (London: Tavistock Publications, 1970); Starhawk, *Dreaming the Dark: Magic, Sex & Politics* (Boston: Beacon Press, 1982); and "The Burning Times," a documentary film produced by Studio D, National Film Board of Canada, which is Part II in the Women and Spirituality series.

4. An interesting side note is that in discussing the homologous nature of men and women's sexual physiognomy, Sharp asserts that women have not one but rather two homologous penises (their vagina and clitoris). For a discussion of this theory, see Laqueur, 14.

5. For a more complete analysis of such cultural inscriptions on women's bodies, see Koehler, 28-107. Also see Ben Barker-Benfield, "Anne Hutchinson and Puritan Attitudes Toward Woman," *Feminist Studies* 1 (Fall 1972): 65-96; and Antonia Fraser, *The Weaker Vessel* (New York: Vintage Books, 1984).

6. A more detailed account of early childbirth rituals is presented in Deborah Kuhn McGregor, "'Childbirth-Travells' and 'Spiritual Estates': Anne Hutchinson and Colonial Boston, 1634-1638," *Caduceus* 5 (Winter 1989): 1-33; and Adrian Wilson, "Participant or Patient: Seventeenth-Century Childbirth from a Mother's Point of View," in *Patients and Practitioners: Lay Perceptions of Medicine in Pre-Industrial Society,* ed. Roy Porter (Cambridge: Cambridge UP, 1985), 129-44.

7. Further studies on "monstrous births" include Patricia Crawford, "Attitudes to Menstruation in Sixteenth- and Seventeenth-Century England," *Past and Present* 91 (May 1981): 47-73; Katharine Park and Lorraine J. Daston, "Unnatural Conceptions: The Study of Monsters in Sixteenth- and Seventeenth-Century France and England," *Past and Present* 92 (August 1981): 20-54; Johan Winsser, "Mary Dyer and the 'Monster' Story," *Quaker History* 79 (Spring 1990): 20-34; and Anne Jacobson Schutte, "'Such Monstrous Births': A Neglected Aspect of the Antinomian Controversy," *Renaissance Quarterly* 38.1 (1985): 85-106.

8. Some of these photographs are included in Martin's study, *The Woman in the Body.* Michael Odent has written a book about his work and hospital, titled *Birth Reborn* (New York: Pantheon, 1984); a second edition is from Medford: Birthworks, 1994. Also see Ina May Gaskin, *Spiritual Midwifery,* 3rd ed. (Summertown, TN: Book Publishing, 1990).

9. There is a great deal of recent scholarship on this work, such as Charlene Spretnak, ed., *The Politics of Women's Spirituality: Essays on the Rise of Spiritual Power within the Feminist Movement* (Garden City: Anchor/Doubleday, 1982); and Christine Downing, *The Goddess: Mythological Images of the Feminine* (New York: Crossroad, 1984).

10. See Gail Patterson Corrington, "The Milk of Salvation: Redemption by the Mother in Late Antiquity and Early Christianity," *Harvard Theological Review* 82 (4): 393-421; and V. Tran Tam Tinh, *Isis Lactans: Corpus des Monuments Greco-Romains d'Isis Allaitant Harpocrate* (Leiden: E. J. Brill 1973).

11. In approaching these various studies, I would suggest the work of Nancy Chodorow in *The Reproduction of Mothering: Psychoanalysis and the Sociology of Gender* (Berkeley: U of California P, 1978); Edie Farwell and Anne Hubbell Maiden, "The Wisdom of Tibetan Childbirth," in *In Context* 31 (1992): 26-31; and Margaret R. Miles, *Carnal Knowing: Female Nakedness and Religious Meaning in the Christian West* (Boston: Beacon Press, 1989).

Works Cited

Beldecos, Athena, et al. "The Importance of Feminist Critique for Contemporary Cell Biology." *Hypatia* 3 (Spring 1988): 61-76.

Berger, Pamela. *The Goddess Obscured: Transformation of the Grain Protectress from Goddess to Saint.* Boston: Beacon, 1985.

Bigwood, Carol. *Earth Muse: Feminism, Nature, and Art.* Philadelphia: Temple UP, 1993.

Bynum, Caroline Walker. "The Female Body and Religious Practice in the Later Middle Ages." In *Fragments for a History of the Human Body, Part I.* Ed. Michel Feher with Ramona Nadaff and Nadia Tazi. New York: Zone Books, 1989.

Christ, Carol P. *Diving Deep and Surfacing: Women Writers on Spiritual Quest.* Boston: Beacon, 1980.

Cixous, Hélène. "The Laugh of the Medusa." In *New French Feminisms.* Eds. Elaine Marks and Isabelle de Courtivron. Amherst: U of Massachusetts P, 1980. 245-64.

Cooey, Paula M. *Religious Imagination and the Body: A Feminist Analysis.* New York: Oxford UP, 1994.

Cosslett, Tess. *Women Writing Childbirth: Modern Discourses of Motherhood.* Manchester: Manchester UP, 1994.

Douglas, Mary. *Purity and Danger: An Analysis of Concepts of Pollution and Taboo.* Harmondsworth, Middlesex, England: Penguin, 1966.

Friedman, Susan Stanford. "Creativity and the Childbirth Metaphor: Gender Difference in Literary Discourse." In *Speaking of Gender.* Ed. Elaine Showalter. New York: Routledge, 1989.

Ganong, William F. *Review of Medical Physiology.* 12th ed. Los Altos, CA: Lange, 1985,

Gimbutas, Marija. *The Language of the Goddess: Unearthing the Hidden Symbols of Western Civilization.* San Francisco: HarperCollins, 1991.

Harvey, William. *Anatomical Excitations Concerning the Generation of Living Creatures.* London: Rancis Leach for Richard Lowndes, 1653.

Kahn, Robbie Pfeufer. *Bearing Meaning: The Language of Birth.* Urbana: U of Illinois P, 1995.

Koehler, Lyle. *A Search for Power: The 'Weaker Sex' in Seventeenth-Century New England.* Urbana: U of Illinois P, 1980.

Kramer, Heinrich, and James Sprenger. *The Malleus Maleficarum.* Trans. Rev. Montague Summers. New York: Dover, 1971.

Kroll, Una. "A Womb-Centred Life." In *Sex and God: Some Varieties of Women's Religious Experience.* Ed. Linda Hurcombe. New York: Routledge and Kegan Paul, 1987.

Laqueur, Thomas. "Orgasm, Generation, and the Politics of Reproductive Biology." In *The Making of the Modern Body: Sexuality and Society in the Nineteenth Century*. Ed. Catherine Gallagher and Thomas Laqueur. Berkeley: U of California P, 1987.

Lerner, Gerda. *The Creation of Patriarchy*. New York: Oxford UP, 1986.

Martin, Emily. *The Woman in the Body: A Cultural Analysis of Reproduction*. Boston: Beacon, 1992.

Mather, Cotton. "A Father Departing . . ." Boston 1723.

Morgan, Robin. *The Anatomy of Freedom: Feminism, Physics, and Global Politics*. New York: Doubleday, 1984.

O'Brien, Mary. *The Politics of Reproduction*. Boston: Routledge and Kegan Paul, 1983.

Odent, Michael. *Birth Reborn*. 2nd ed. Medford: Birthworks, 1994.

Olds, Sharon. "The Language of the Brag." *Satan Says*. Pittsburgh: U of Pittsburgh P, 1980. 44-45.

Rabuzzi, Kathryn Allen. *Mother With Child: Transformations Through Childbirth*. Bloomington: Indiana UP, 1994.

Rich, Adrienne. *Of Woman Born: Motherhood as Experience and Institution*. New York: Bantam, 1976.

Rothman, Barbara Katz. *In Labor: Women and Power in the Birthplace*. New York: W. W. Norton, 1982.

Shange, Ntozake. *Nappy Edges*. New York: Bantam, 1978.

Sharp, Jane. *The Midwives Book, or the Whole Art of Midwifery Discovered, Directing Childbearing Women How to Behave Themselves in Their Conception, Breeding, Bearing, and Nursing of Children*. London: Simon Miller, 1671.

Warner, Marina. *Alone of All Her Sex: The Myth and Cult of the Virgin Mary*. New York: Pocket Books, 1976.

3

CLAIMING OUR BIRTH-WRITE:
THE POETRY OF AMERICAN MOTHERS

Susan MacCallum-Whitcomb

Anne Bradstreet, America's first poet, has garnered praise as both a colonial writer and as a woman writer. But it should be remembered that she was a literary mother as well, and that through her American maternity poetry had an auspicious start. Motherhood, for Bradstreet, was a defining experience. In her poems, she speaks of the "labor," "pain," "cost," and "care" that child-rearing requires (184); yet she values the knowledge gained from maternity enough to make use of it not only in her domestic pieces but also in more doctrinaire works such as "The Four Ages of Man." Indeed, maternity permeates Bradstreet's thinking to such an extent that her other great loves, her God, her husband, and her writing, can all be defined in terms of it.[1]

The fact that she was a mother was, in short, important to Bradstreet, and it has also been important to a great many of her readers. Adrienne Rich, for one, has admitted that she was initially attracted to Bradstreet because "she was one of the few women writers I knew anything about who had also been a mother" (21). Of course, Rich's admiration was not based on this alone: in her article "The Tensions of Anne Bradstreet" both the elder poet's talent and tenacity are given special mention. "To have written poems, the first good poems in America, while rearing eight children, lying frequently sick, keeping house at the edge of wilderness," Rich concludes, "was to have managed a poet's range and extension within confines as severe as any American poet has confronted" (32).

Rich's high regard for Bradstreet's work is certainly warranted. Her work represents a great achievement. But, in the context of American maternity poetry, the argument regarding the severity of Bradstreet's circumstances is not wholly convincing. Rich, for example, begins with the business of rearing children. This did pose difficulties: Bradstreet's poems, after all, were "the fruit but of some few hours, curtailed from her sleep, and other refreshments" (Bradstreet 526).[2] However, issues of occupation and interruption continue to jeopardize the literary production of mothers, as contemporary pieces like Susan Griffin's "This Is the Story of the Day in the Life of a Woman Trying" and Marilyn Nelson Waniek's "Levitation with Baby" make abundantly clear. In fact, poems on these themes are so common that they comprise a whole sub-genre in American maternity poetry. Simply put, the obligations which come with child-raising did not change substantially from Bradstreet's time to our own. Other things did, and not necessarily for the better.

Rich goes on to cite the inherent dangers and difficulties of Bradstreet's frontier existence;[3] but according to Pattie Cowell, "students of colonial history have demonstrated the relative advantages possessed by American women [in this period] in comparison with their British peers, and even in comparison with nineteenth century American women" (7). One such advantage was the importance attached to the family in colonial communities. Puritan society, for instance, was modelled on the family, and "all power" in it "derived from the family unit." Therefore, everything related to the creation of the family was considered significant. On a practical level, this meant that child-bearing (at least within the context of marriage) was viewed as more than simply a worthwhile endeavour: it was elevated to the level of a sacred "duty" (Walker 10-11). From the poet's perspective, this also meant that family life, the life mothers knew so intimately, was accepted as being worthy of literary treatment.

The emphasis placed on religion in these communities gave writers like Bradstreet further legitimacy.[4] Because the Puritans' over-riding concern with spiritual matters, coupled with their penchant for introspection, created an environment in which the internal was valued over the external, the literary mothers' lack of worldly experience did not, for once, prove to be a liability. Since God's handiwork was everywhere in evidence even the domestic sphere was able to furnish the necessary examples of his grace and goodness.

Cowell goes on to argue that "the religious base of colonial life, particularly in Puritan and Quaker societies, assured women of spiritual (if not practical) equality, providing the theological sanction for the inherent value of women's lives regardless of their subordinate function" (6).[5] This, by extension, also allowed for a degree of artistic equality because it "created similar preoccupations" for both male and female writers. As a result, common "themes predominate among seventeenth century women as among men' " (17).

For proof of this, we need only compare the works of Anne Bradstreet with those of Edward Taylor, her only peer in early American poetry. Both are clearly cut from the same "homespun cloth" (Bradstreet 178). Bradstreet, for instance, shared his interest in spiritual matters and, as poems such as "Housewifery" and "Upon Wedlock and Death of Children" indicate, Taylor shared her concern with domestic and familial living. Thus while Anne Bradstreet was expected to attend to "such things as belong to women" and stay firmly "in the place God had set her" (Winthrop 225), she could, at least, find there suitable material for poetry. And that poetry, in turn, could win her the admiration, not only of family members and fellow writers, but of leading religious figures such as Cotton Mather as well.[6]

In the final accounting, then, life "at the edge of the wilderness" (Rich 32) was in many respects preferable to the ghetto (literary or otherwise) that Bradstreet's descendants were often forced to live in. Admittedly, Bradstreet was not representative of all women in her era: only her social standing, and the attendant economic and educational advantages she enjoyed, enabled her to write at all. Similarly, the type of writing she engaged in only became privileged discourse because her male contemporaries deemed it so. Nonetheless, Bradstreet was able to write as a mother and to incorporate her child-rearing and home-making experiences into her work. Other pre-revolutionary poets such as Jane Colman Turell, Martha Brewster, Judith Sargent Murray, Ann Eliza Bleecker, and Sarah Wentworth Morton were able to do the same.

Changing circumstances, however, eventually caused the sanction for domestic writing to be revoked. Long after the religious focus of colonial life began to decline, the family home continued to be viewed in a positive light, (and so continued to be regarded as an appropriate subject for literature), due to the physical, economic, and psychological security it represented. But during the five decades which followed the end of the War of Independence, American society was radically altered, and the perceived value of the family home was greatly diminished. In this period, as Nancy Cott writes, a variety of social, political, and economic factors conspired to divert the focus of American life away from the domestic realm:

Trends such as the decline of traditional determinants of deference, the assertion of an individualist ethos, increasing extremes of wealth and poverty, and replacement of unitary association networks by pluralistic ones, indicated deep change in social relations. Differentiation and specialization characterized this transformation of society. These were portrayed and symbolized most powerfully in the separation of production and exchange from the domestic arena— the division between "world" and "home." (66-67, cf 3)

Emphasis, in other words, began to be placed on the individual rather than the familial: the factory and marketplace began to take precedence over the hearth and field. So the "home" (which had hitherto been viewed as the centre of attention and activity) soon came to be seen as a separate entity, isolated from the burgeoning "world" around it. Since women, bound by a host of societal injunctions, clearly belonged in the former and men belonged to the latter, the difference in their assigned roles became increasingly clear.

For mothers, especially those with literary aspirations, the consequences were devastating. While they remained immobile, the menfolk were drawn "away from the household, abbreviating their presence in the family and their roles in child-rearing" (Cott 46). In the process, the common ground poetic parents once shared was lost, and their paths diverged. Fathers were able, indeed encouraged, to venture off on the road "less travelled" (Frost 72). Mothers, meanwhile, were left home to knit booties and talk amongst themselves.

We can find ample evidence of this change in the simultaneous development of two distinct literary traditions. On one hand, there were the great works of the American Renaissance: "important" works produced by men. On the other was the mass of women's writing arising out of the cult of domesticity which Nathaniel Hawthorne blithely dismissed as the "trash" produced by a "d----d mob of scribbling women" (304).

Hawthorne's use of the term "mob" is accurate in some respects, for women and, more specifically, mothers, still wrote in the nineteenth century: indeed some wrote voluminously. But if these "detestable," "ink-stained women" (Hawthorne 161) wished to publish, the range of tones and subjects available to them was relatively narrow. Their inspiration, as Caroline May wrote approvingly in her introduction to *The American Female Poets* (1848), was expected to come from the "heart," not the "head," and their themes were to be "derived from the incidents and associations of every-day life," from the "home, with its quiet joys, its deep pure sympathies, and its secret sorrows" (vi). Unfortunately, May's views were widely held. The editors of magazines such as *Godey's, Graham's,* and *Lady's Wreath,* for example, "published and applauded sentimentality." In the poems found within their pages

. . . the sentimental is less a matter of self-dramatization (although that does occur) than a reliance on words like "sweet" and "the thorn," an over-fondness for idealizing children or the dead, a tendency to take comfort in simplistic conceptions of life and pious platitudes . . . [T]hese poems are a manifestation of the fact that women were powerless and so deeply trapped in their own powerlessness that they were afraid to disappoint the very critical expectations that kept them mired in mediocrity. (Walker 57)

As women writing "pinched and narrow" works (Emerson 402)[7] addressed largely to other women, the nineteenth century poetesses could only achieve popular success. Serious critical consideration was reserved for men speaking to men about topics which were assumed to be of significance to the world at large, and in this era of fervent nationalism no topic was more important than America itself.

In 1844 Ralph Waldo Emerson maintained that "America is a poem in our eyes" (238), and Walt Whitman concurred when he wrote that the "United States themselves are essentially the greatest poem" (411). Both men also agreed that American poetry should reflect this seemingly simple fact by emphasizing the country's "ample geography," "incomparable materials" (Emerson 238), and "enormous diversity" (Whitman 413). Hence, prospective poets were asked "Who are you indeed who would talk or sing to America? Have you studied out the land, its idioms and men?" (Whitman 247), and for American mothers the answer was invariably "no."

The criteria for the great American poem quickly was set; the job description for the "true" American poet was written; and the marginalization of those who were either unwilling or unable to conform to the rigid, new standards became inevitable. For American women in general, the insistence on a male model, grounded by definition in alien experiences, made the writing of poetry very difficult. For American mothers, women bound by an even wider range of physical and cultural imperatives, the task was more difficult still.

We can see just how formidable the injunctions were against mothers who aspired to be poets (as opposed to poetesses) if we look more closely at the works of Emerson and Whitman. The former described the American poet as "the complete man" (223), "the winged man" (226), "the man of Beauty" (223). If generous allowance is made for his non-inclusive langauge, Emerson's vision of the poet might be extended to include women without children; however, his corollary that the poet must also be "the man without impediment" (224) firmly excluded mothers because it demanded a freedom from responsibility which they had traditionally been denied. To create poetic works, Emerson argued, the poet must begin by "unlocking, at all risks, his human doors" (233): no small feat for the woman who must baby-proof the house, stock the nursery and arrange for appropriate child-care before she unlocks even the door to her own dwelling. To be "struck with poetic wonder," Emerson decreed, the poet must "leave far behind all human relations, wife, mother and child, and live only with the savages—water, air, light, carbon, lime, and granite" (88). This is an impossible feat for the mother who would have to escape from her children and then somehow manage to escape from herself.

Emerson upheld a distinctly male model of experience. Interpreting literally the national dream of life, liberty and the pursuit of happiness, he celebrated the wholly unencumbered man who could "traverse the whole scale of experience" (224). And while his living embodiment of the American dream embarked on a life of "rambling" (225), recording his experiences in "spermatic, prophesying, man-making words" (Emerson, qtd. in Leverenz 39), the mother was left bound and gagged in a "jailyard of individual relations" (234). Indeed, as far as Emerson was concerned, this jailyard seemed the best place for her, because mothers, in his estimation, were not only incapable of creativity themselves, they were obstacles to male creativity as well. In other words, they were fit to be neither poet nor muse. Household chores and private responsibilities "untune and disqualify me for writing," Emerson argued: "I think then the writer ought not to be married, ought not to have a family" (420).[8]

The difficult situation literary mothers found themselves in as a result was further exacerbated by Whitman, that legendary ejaculator greeted by Emerson at the "beginning of a great career" (362). Like Emerson, Whitman saw the American poet as a male figure. "His spirit," Whitman wrote in the preface to the 1855 edition of *Leaves of Grass,* "responds to his country's spirit . . . he incarnates its geography and natural life and rivers and lakes" (412). To accomplish this task, Whitman's archetypal poet once again was required to be a "man without impediment" (Emerson 224), able not only to "lean and loafe at [his] ease" (25) but to "tramp a perpetual journey" (63). Freedom and mobility, therefore, remained central to his definition of the poet. In Whitman's view, the poet had to "Unscrew the locks from the doors!/Unscrew the doors themselves from their jambs!" (41) because "heroic deeds were all conceiv'd in the open air, and all free poems also" (109). Mothers, trapped in their "shutter'd room" (65) due to a different sort of conception, were left metaphorically barren. But even if mothers had been able to conceive poems, they could not have brought them to term. Producing the "gigantic and generous" (412) works that Whitman called for required both a great deal of energy and long stretches of uninterrupted writing time: simply put, it required the kind of commitment that only a "childless, lonely old grubber" (Ginsberg 29) like Whitman himself could make.

Emerson's attitude toward the literary mother is troublesome enough; however, in Whitman's case the problem is compounded by his pretence of inclusivity. Although Whitman insisted that "the mother . . . is every bit as much as the father" (156), his sentimental portrayal of her belies this claim. The mother described by Whitman has a "benignant" (344) face "illuminated" (323) by "beautiful maternal cares" (306). She does the "cooking, washing, child-nursing, house-tending—she beams sunshine out of all these duties and makes them illustrious" (483). She is curiously conventional. She is also conspicuously quiet. We hear the "mother's voice in lullaby or hymn" (284), we hear her speak with "mild words" (258), but never does she sound a "barbaric yawp" (68). One could attribute the mother's muted tones to practicality: she may simply not wish to disturb the babe that Whitman invariably shows either at the breast endlessly nursing or in "the cradle endlessly rocking" (180). But it is more likely that Whitman, in his desire to be the conduit through which "long dumb voices" resound (41), does not want her to speak for herself.[9]

If women held out any hope of using their own voices and gaining serious literary consideration in a phallocentric society, it was necessary for them to free themselves from as many female responsibilities as possible. Historically, this meant that American women were forced to make a choice. They could forgo child-bearing to dedicate themselves to their art, and, in doing so, risk being dismissed as aberrations; or they could have children, settle into a domestic routine, and give up their poetic aspirations.

Some women, like the nineteenth century poet Lucretia Davidson, consciously chose the first option. According to her mother, Davidson felt that she "could not do justice to husband or children, while her whole soul was absorbed in literary pursuits; she was not willing to resign them for any man, therefore, she had formed the resolution to lead a single life" (qtd. in Walker 75). Early in this century, Sara Teasdale made a similar decision when she aborted a fetus because, in the words of Elaine Showalter, she was "unable to imagine maternity and poetic creativity as other than antagonistic roles" (110). Others, like Alice Williams Brotherton, chose a different path. "I thought to win me a name," Brotherton writes, that would "ring in the ear of the world—/ [But] How can I work with small pink fists/About my fingers curled? (76). Feeling unequal to the challenge, Brotherton bids "adieu to name and to fame" (76). We will never know how many other literary mothers were forced to do the same.

Certainly there must have been many, for when Amy Lowell wrote "The Sisters" in 1925 the ability of any woman to combine motherhood with a writing career still seemed "miraculous" (459). Lowell, however, did feel that women were potentially "double-bearing,/With matrices in body and in brain" (459), and in her lifetime this belief was beginning to be put into practice through the creation of an alternative model for poetry based on female experience: one which not only allowed for the possibility of motherhood, but recognized it as asset rather than an artistic liability.

Obstacles remained and still remain today. After all, mothers continue to deal with the reality of child-rearing and all of its relentless demands. Moreover, as poems such as Cynthia MacDonald's "Instruction from Bly" and Alicia Ostriker's "Propaganda Poem" reveal, the "carping tongue" which Anne Bradstreet complained of (7) has never really been silenced: women poets must still contend with the admonishment of their peers, male and female alike. Nevertheless, America's literary mothers in the twentieth century have regained confidence in their creative powers, both poetic and reproductive.[10]

Power itself has become a central theme for many of them. Maternal figures, for example, often recast themselves in powerful roles. Moving beyond the stereotypes of the romanticized martyr or Madonna, they describe themselves as providers or protectors. In doing so, they not only reverse traditional expectations of the passive, dependent mother; they also succeed in reducing the importance of the father by effectively usurping the positions from which his authority is typically derived. Of course, male poets had set the precedent for this. Emerson expropriated the mother's power by describing his own creativity in terms of gestation and birth.[11] Whitman, furthermore, expropriated the mother's voice when he claimed, "The Female equally with the Male I sing" (5), the "Maternal as well as Paternal" (36); and he assumed (or rather consumed) her persona entirely when he insisted, "I am the most venerable mother" (132). So it is not surprising that mothers would engage in some expropriation of their own when the opportunity arose.

But a number of them go further still: rather than dealing with generic fathers, they challenge, with varying degrees of directness, the fathers of American poetry. These women subvert the phallocentric national model by taking the words of its primary promoters (especially Whitman's because of the durability of his reputation and the influence he exerted on successive generations of American poets) and applying them to maternal experience. In the process, they prove that mothers are not just capable of writing poetry, they are as well qualified to write it as the icons of the American literary tradition.

One such woman was Mina Loy who in 1923 published "Parturition:" a "lascivious revelation" (69) which was considered obscene when it first appeared, and which remains, arguably, the most vivid portrayal of labor and delivery in American maternity poetry. In literature, the strenuous physical and mental activity required to produce a child had long been underestimated: Whitman, for one, described a "sacred parturition scene" in which a "happy painless mother birth'd a perfect child" (269). And to such treatments, Loy's "Parturition" offers a welcome corrective.

Loy steadfastly refused to sentimentalize (and thereby trivialize) the exhausting "struggle" (67) which made a woman into a mother. Instead she borrowed Whitman's vocabulary, whether intentionally or not, translating both his words and his wandering in terms of her own birthing experience. "I am the centre/Of a circle of pain," Loy writes, the centre of a "congested cosmos" (67, cf Whitman 41). "I am climbing a distorted mountain of agony/. . . I must traverse/Traversing myself" (68). Here Loy does in metaphor what Whitman does in fact, but in other instances the reverse is true.

Whitman, for example, had aspired to live in harmony with Nature: through maternity, Loy actually becomes one with it by identifying with the "feathered moth" (69), speaking with the voice of the "wild beast" (68), and merging into cat and insect alike. Similarly, Whitman could only claim to "have the best of time and space" (63). Loy, on the other hand, contains all time and all space, because in pregnancy she "races/Through the subliminal deposits of evolutionary/processes" (69) while the "Stir of incipient life" precipitates into her the "contents of the universe" (70). And the poet asserts that she, not a man like Whitman, is truly "the most venerable mother" (132), boasting:

> Mother I am
> Identical
> With infinite Maternity
> Indivisible
> Acutely
> I am absorbed
> Into
> The was-is-ever-shall-be
> Of cosmic reproductivity. (70)

As these lines demonstrate, even Loy's formal innovations can be taken as a challenge to Whitman. In comparing the works of the two poets, Carolyn Burke rightly contends that Loy "had to revise his song of the (male) self to suit a female subject." After citing as an example Whitman's expansive lines, Burke explains that "Loy, by contrast, worked out a compact, compressed free verse line that could simulate the rhythmic contractions and expansions of labor. At the same time she approached the blank page as if it were a canvas: a visual medium in which to recreate the inner spaces of the female body" (53). Since Whitman maintained that "In the best poems re-appears the body, man's or woman's, well-shaped, natural" (161), it would seem that Loy once again succeeds at doing "that which others dream of" (Emerson 224).

Mina Loy, as "Parturition" forcefully illustrates, did not accept the popular notion that a woman could not be a mother and a poet: "Every woman," she argued, had "a right to maternity" (270). Loy believed that "Nature endowed the Complete Woman with a faculty for expressing herself through all her functions" (270), and many of the American women poets who followed her have agreed. Anne Sexton, who persistently wrote out of female experience, subverting patriarchal tradition along the way, is only one example.

Like Loy, Sexton issued an implicit challenge to Whitman in a number of her poems. "The Civil War," for instance, is an abbreviated version of "a song of myself" (Sexton 419), while "In Celebration of My Uterus" is an anthem for herself and her sisters. As the title of this latter work suggests, Sexton's intent is to celebrate the maternal (or at least the potentially maternal). But by making use of the repetitive sentence structures so familiar to Whitman's readers, she appears to also be offering a feminist reply to the elder poet's song of the "phallus" (69). In the idyllic world which Sexton creates—a world from which men are notably absent—she defines herself as a whole being. She has a "soul," for instance, as well as a body (182): and in valorizing "the woman I am" (182), she proves that she has a firm sense of both her identity and her own creative potential. Most importantly, she emphasizes her voice and hears it echoed in women "everywhere," all of whom "seem to be singing, although some can not/sing a note" (182).

"In Celebration of My Uterus" is, as Richard Morton has noted, "essentially political: hymning the vitality of the woman's body, and cataloguing the joyous singing of women in all places and times, it achieves a Whitmanesque force and conviction (65). The same can be said of her psalm sequence "Oh Ye Tongues," which can be read as a variation on Whitman's "great psalm of the republic" (413). For our purposes, this last work is the most significant. In it Sexton makes use of the parallel constructions, biblical phrasing and oracular tone which had become so strongly identified with Whitman's work. Moreover, like him, she shifts her focus frequently, moving from the particular to the general, from discussions of her own life to ruminations about life in America. Yet unlike Whitman, Sexton does not presume to speak for everyone. She speaks as a woman, and, in doing so, gives a credibility to woman's experiences (specifically those associated with pregnancy and child-rearing) which Whitman would have found inconceivable.

Issues of maternity are first addressed in "Eighth Psalm," where the pregnancy of Sexton's speaker is made apparent. In the earlier psalms, she had employed images of confinement and oppression to define her life. Her childhood was a "Jail," a box-like room with "Four thick walls," and a "low menacing ceiling." Her house, even her country, was "only this room" and "Anne" was "locked in" it (402-06). Yet when she turns to the adult role of mother a different attitude emerges, for the birth of her child puts an end to the speaker's "confinement" both literally and figuratively (409). She now can "walk through" "many worlds" (409) and "master" many "mountains" (412).

For Sexton, in other words, maternity liberates rather than binds, and through it her speaker is transformed from a passive agent into a powerful one. The child who had been exploited is now perceived as a woman who is "dangerous" (408). The child who felt so alienated that she could only refer to her imprisoned self in the third person has become a mature woman who can say with conviction "*I* am not locked up" (411, emphasis mine). The child who once felt so lonely, so insignificant that she had to create an "imaginary brother" for "company" and completion (401-02) can now rejoice that "she is a magnitude, she is many" (408).

Here Sexton echoes Whitman's famous line from "Song of Myself": "(I am large, I contain multitudes)" (68). However, the context of Sexton's poem makes clear that her speaker's claim is more valid than his because it is true in the physical as well as the metaphoric sense. Not only does she carry the child within her (and thereby embody even Whitman's brackets), she also carries Christopher, the child's father, because he is a product of her imagination. The mother proves that she is "an acme of things accomplish'd" and "an encloser of things to be" (Whitman 62).

Sharon Olds' birth poem "The Language of the Brag" offers yet another challenge to Whitman's authority. "I have wanted some epic use for my excellent body," Olds writes:

> some heroism, some American achievement
> beyond the ordinary for my extraordinary self,
> magnetic and tensile, I have stood by the sandlot
> and watched the boys play.
> I have wanted courage, I have thought about fire
> and the crossing of waterfalls . . . (44)

But rather than trying to fit herself into a masculine paradigm, Olds chooses maternity. Whitman had already envisioned just such a woman. He had dreamed of begetting "fierce and athletic girls" (77), a whole "race of perfect Mothers" who would distinguish themselves through their fecundity (463). What he did not take into account was that the power they derived from motherhood would ultimately pose a threat to his own.

Despite the praise Whitman lavishes on "sane athletic maternity" (463), he often describes mothers as passively receptive vessels. We see this most clearly in "A Woman Waits for Me" from "Children of Adam:"[12]

> It is I, you women, I make my way,
> I am stern, acrid, large, undissuadable, but I love you,
> I do not hurt you any more than is necessary for you,
> I pour the stuff to start sons and daughters fit for these States,
> I press with slow rude muscle,
> I brace myself effectually, I listen to no entreaties,
> I dare not withdraw till I deposit what has so long accumulated within me.
> Through you I drain the pent-up rivers of myself . . . (77)

Here the emphasis is placed firmly on the father. Here only his "slow rude muscle" is put to use. But Olds, speaking with "perfect personal candor" (Whitman 422), turns attention to her own "electric muscles" (Olds 44, cf Whitman 70). In fact, no father is ever mentioned in "The Language of the Brag." In the poems discussed above the paternal role had steadily declined: Loy spoke of a real, yet distant, father and Sexton named as father an imaginary man she herself created. Olds, in turn, manages to circumvent the question of paternity altogether by becoming essentially self-generating. So even the biological function of the father is rendered metaphorically obsolete. The male presence vanishes and maternal power is confirmed.

The legitimacy of the maternal voice is confirmed as well. Believing that women's "crowning attribute" (462) was producing babies (the pun is probably unintentional), Whitman had made them virtually mute. But Olds shows that "the exclamations of women taken suddenly who hurry home and give birth to babes" need no longer be "howls restrain'd by decorum" (Whitman 30). She speaks for herself, defiantly celebrating motherhood and demanding that her accomplishment be recognized:

> I have done what you wanted to do, Walt Whitman,
> Allen Ginsberg, I have done this thing,
> I and the other women this exceptional
> act with the exceptional heroic body,
> this giving birth . . . (45)

Olds indeed does what Whitman and his kind "wanted to do," what they could only talk about doing. Whitman "chant[s] the chant of dilation" (39): Olds, in labor, is dilated. Whitman sings "the song of procreation" (69): Olds actually procreates. Whitman writes that he "will make the poems of my body" (17): Olds makes poems out of her body. Hers is the "language of blood," the poetry of the "glistening verb" (44), and through it she puts her "proud American boast/right here with the others" (45).

The boasts made by Olds, Sexton, and Loy all validate the maternal experience and prove how well-suited mothers are to write about "Life immense in passion, pulse, and power (Whitman 5). Like Emerson and others, Walt Whitman underestimated the mother's voice when he distinguished between those who could "perceive" and "tell" and those who could "conceive children and bring them up well" (420). However, American maternity poetry as a whole reveals that he was right in one regard: "Births have brought us richness and variety,/And other births will bring us richness and variety" as well (61).

Notes

1. Simon Bradstreet, for example, is identified not only as the poet's husband but as the father of her children, and in "Before the Birth of One of Her Children" the poet focuses specifically on this latter role. In "Meditations Divine and Morall," Bradstreet compares God with both a nursing mother and a "prudent mother" (200). In "The Author to Her Book," she uses an extended metaphor, describing her poetry as a "rambling brat," the "ill-form'd offspring" of her "feeble brain" (177).

2. The same could be said for other pre-revolutionary literary mothers. Ann Eliza Bleecker, for example, lamented that ". . . Amidst domestic cares to rhyme/I find no pleasure, and I find no time," and Sarah Wentworth Morton set the Muses' "enchantment" against the "personal occupation, which my station renders obligatory . . ." (qtd. in Cowell 5, 11-12).

3. Rich also points to the fact that Bradstreet was "lying frequently sick" (32), but many would argue that this was still better than being forced into the role of "barbiturate-drenched Camilles/With continuous periods, murmuring softly on sofas" and occasionally vomiting up the "sickly effluvium" that later passed for women's poetry (Kizer 171).

4. Despite the stereotypical perception of the Puritan faith, the editors of Bradstreet's *Complete Works* contend that "her society was less repressive in its attitude toward women than we imagine. After all, Bradstreet was *not* censured, disciplined, or in any way ostracized for her art, thought, or personal assertiveness so far as we know. Rather she was praised and encouraged" (xiii).

5. Although she remains sympathetic to the plight of colonial women, Cowell is not blind to the benefits they enjoyed. She adds, for instance, that

their "economic value" was heightened because of chronic "labor shortages," and that "favourable sex ratios" also worked to their advantage. (6)

6. *The Tenth Muse,* of course, was first published on the initiative of her brother-in-law, Rev. John Woodbridge, and Bradstreet's manuscript books were carefully preserved by her son Simon (Bradstreet xxi). Edward Taylor owned a copy of her verses: indeed, in the introduction to Taylor's *Poetical Works,* Thomas H. Johnson points out that, "oddly enough," it was the "only one book of English poetry" in his collection (19). Finally, in *Magnalia Christi Americana,* Mather praised her work as "a monument for her memory beyond the stateliest marbles" (II, 233).

7. Emerson used this phrase when criticizing the works of Jane Austen; however, it could be applied just as easily to the literature produced by his own country-women.

8. This particular quote is taken from *The Journals and Miscellaneous Notebooks of Ralph Waldo Emerson.* Unless otherwise noted, all other quotes from Emerson's work are taken from *Selections from Ralph Waldo Emerson: An Organic Anthology.* (Cf. the journal entry for May, 1859 in *Selections,* 376.)

9. This belief is reinforced by Whitman's comment in the Brooklyn *Daily Times* (July 9, 1857): "The Majority of people do not want their daughters trained to become authoresses and poets. We want a race of women turned out from our schools, not of pedants and bluestockings. One genuine woman is worth a dozen Fanny Ferns" (qtd. in Kaplan 225).

10. A short list of those American women who have been able not only to produce poetry but to use their poetry to reflect and validate maternal experience would include Louise Bogan, Gwendolyn Brooks, Lucille Clifton, Babette Deutsch, Rita Dove, Susan Griffin, Marilyn Hacker, Maxine Kumin, Denise Levertov, Mina Loy, Sandra McPherson, Sharon Olds, Alicia Ostriker, Linda Pastan, Sylvia Plath, Muriel Rukeyser, Adrienne Rich, Anne Sexton, Genevieve Taggard, and Marilyn Nelson Waniek.

11. Emerson contends that once "the soul of the poet has come to ripeness of thought" its poems or "progeny" detach and pass away from "their mortal parent" to become independent and "vivacious offspring" (232).

12. The titles themselves reflect his attitude: note the passive verb of the former and the possessive form of the latter.

Works Cited

Bradstreet, Anne. *The Complete Works of Anne Bradstreet.* Eds. Joseph R. McElrath, Jr., and Allan P. Robb. Boston: Twayne, 1981.

Brotherton, Alice Williams. "Woman and Artist." *Mother-Song and Child-Song.* Ed. Charlotte Brewster Jordan. New York: Stokes, 1898. 76.

Burke, Carolyn. "The New Poetry and the New Woman:" Mina Loy." *Coming to Light: American Women Poets in the Twentieth Century.* Ed. Diane Wood Middlebrook and Marilyn Yalom. Ann Arbor: U of Michigan P, 1985. 37-57.

Cott, Nancy F. *The Bonds of Womanhood: "Woman's Sphere" in New England, 1780-1835.* New Haven: Yale UP, 1977.

Cowell, Pattie, ed. *Women Poets in Pre-Revolutionary America, 1650-1775: An Anthology.* Troy: Whitston, 1981.

Emerson, Ralph Waldo. *The Journals and Miscellaneous Notebooks of Ralph Waldo Emerson.* Vol. VII, 1838-1842. Ed. A. W. Plumstead and Harrison Hayford. Cambridge: Belknap-Harvard, 1969.

——, Ralph Waldo. *Selections from Ralph Waldo Emerson: An Organic Anthology.* Ed. Stephen E. Whicher. Boston: Houghton Mifflin, 1957.

Frost, Robert. "The Road Not Taken." *Selected Poems of Robert Frost.* New York: Holt, Rinehart and Winston, 1963. 71-72.

Ginsberg, Allen. "A Supermarket in California." *"Howl" and Other Poems.* San Francisco: City Lights, 1993. 29-30.

Hawthorne, Nathaniel. *The Letters, 1853-1856.* Eds. Thomas Woodson et al. Columbus: Ohio State UP, 1987.

Kaplan, Justin. *Walt Whitman: A Life.* New York: Simon and Schuster, 1980.

Kizer, Carolyn. "Pro Femina." *No More Masks!: An Anthology of Twentieth-Century American Women Poets.* Ed. Florence Howe. New York: Harper Perennial, 1993. 169-72.

Leverenz, David. "The Politics of Emerson's Man-Making Words." *PMLA* 101 (1986): 38-56.

Lowell, Amy. "The Sisters." *The Complete Poetical Works of Amy Lowell.* Boston: Houghton Mifflin, 1955. 459-61.

Loy, Mina. *The Last Lunar Baedeker.* Ed. Roger L. Conover. Highlands, NC: Jargon, 1982.

Mather, Cotton. *Magnalia Christi Americana.* Vol. II. Ed. Kenneth B. Murdock. Cambridge: Harvard UP, 1977.

May, Caroline, ed. *The American Female Poets.* Philadelphia: Lindsay and Blakiston, 1848.

Morton, Richard. *Anne Sexton's Poetry of Redemption: The Chronology of a Pilgrimage.* Lewiston, NY: Edwin Mellon, 1989.

Olds, Sharon. *Satan Says.* Pittsburgh: U of Pittsburgh P, 1980.

Rich, Adrienne. "The Tensions of Anne Bradstreet." *On Lies, Secrets, and Silence: Selected Prose, 1966-1978.* New York: Norton, 1979. 21-32.

Sexton, Anne. *The Complete Poems.* Ed. Linda Gray Sexton. Boston: Houghton Mifflin, 1981.

Showalter, Elaine. *Sister's Choice: Tradition and Change in American Women's Writing.* Oxford: Clarendon P, 1991.

Taylor, Edward. *The Poetical Works of Edward Taylor.* Ed. Thomas H. Johnson. Princeton: Princeton UP, 1966.

Walker, Cheryl. *The Nightingale's Burden: Women Poets and American Culture Before 1900.* Bloomington: Indiana UP, 1982.

Whitman, Walt. *Complete Poetry and Selected Prose.* Ed. James E. Miller, Jr. Boston: Houghton Mifflin, 1959.

Winthrop, John. *Winthrop's Journal: "History of New England," 1630-1649.* Vol. 2. Ed. James Kendall Hosmer. New York: Barnes and Noble, 1959.

4

THIRTY-NINE WEEKS:
PREGNANCY AND BIRTH IMAGERY
IN KATE CHOPIN'S *THE AWAKENING*

Gail Lippincott

Kate Chopin, much like her protagonist Edna Pontellier, "dares and defies" the cultural restrictions, both literary and social, of the nineteenth century as she delicately incorporates pregnancy and birth imagery in her 1899 novel, *The Awakening* (176). For the most part, however, this subtle imagery was unnoticed, and continues to be overlooked, because Chopin so skillfully creates what we now call a double-voiced or double-edged discourse, discourse used to "gain critical recognition from the establishment while at the same time resisting and subverting it" (Schor 267). This essay explores Chopin's second voice, illuminating the hidden emotions and rhythms of pregnancy she has woven into her daring novel. *The Awakening* portrays the literal pregnancy of the character Adele Ratignolle with what Emily Toth calls "the discretion required in the 1890s" based on "the stages of pregnancy she [Chopin] knew so well" (332). In addition, Chopin weaves another pregnancy into her maternal subtext: a closer examination reveals that Edna is also pregnant—metaphorically—with her own individual self. Chopin's strategy foreshadows what Adrienne Rich maintains has become a recurring metaphor for feminist writers, that of giving birth to oneself (156). Employing historical as well as modern childbirth literature and sociological studies, this essay teases out the subtle and apparently deliberate evidence of Edna Pontellier's "pregnancy."

While many modern literary critics perceive that Edna undergoes a metaphoric rebirth at the end of the novel when she strips off her old bathing suit and stands naked "like some new-born creature" (*Awakening* 175), only a few have recognized the language of pregnancy that precedes such a rebirth, a tribute to Chopin's skillful authorship. Cynthia Griffin Wolff, for example, appreciates that Edna, while not pregnant herself, becomes "intensely involved with Adele's pregnancy" in order to recreate the "state of total union" that pregnant women achieve

55

between themselves and the fetus ("Thanatos" 256). Male critic and early biographer Per Seyersted recognizes that the novel "covers two gestations and births"; although he does not apprehend a pregnant Edna, he perceives her "slow birth as a sexual and authentic being, and the counterpointed pregnancy and confinement of Adele" (153). Similarly, Cheryl Jacobsen does not describe a metaphoric pregnancy, but observes the end result when she notes that "Edna's labor is too advanced for [Doctor] Mandelet to be the *accoucher* to her emerging autonomous Self" (123). Toth perceptively discerns that the novel "takes place over the nine months" of Adele's pregnancy (331), while Peggy Skaggs recognizes that "Edna's 'awakening' progresses simultaneously with Adele's pregnancy; thus the structure of the novel is related to the basic, natural rhythm of the human gestation cycle" (89). While these critics catch a glimmer of Chopin's double-edged discourse that captures the moods and materiality of a literal pregnancy, the subtle evocation of Edna's metaphoric pregnancy remains hidden.

Even though frequent pregnancies were the lot of most nineteenth-century married women, domestic fiction novels written by, for, and about these women gloss over this incredibly central part of their lives. As Dale Spender exclaims, "Given the number of novels in which childbirth is of central significance it is staggering to find that the event itself is virtually invisible. Women labour between the lines, children are born outside the pages, and rare even is the record of women's response to such a momentous occasion" (115). Madeleine Riley explains that "the novelists were on their guard to ensure that no charge of immodesty could be made against them" (74). Noting that author Elizabeth Gaskell, a mother herself, includes no details of the many births that occur in her novels, Riley remarks that "new babies are revealed, blandly, in their mothers' beds without explanation as to how they got there" (77). Nothing was written about pregnancy itself, Carole Stone says, because "in Chopin's era childbirth was considered a woman's noblest act; to write of it otherwise was unacceptable. Thus, the clinical details of pregnancy and birthing remained largely unwritten" (23). Chopin is careful not to transgress the bounds of good taste regarding the details of pregnancy and childbirth, although Toth and Heather Kirk Thomas show how she mocks many sentimental conventions of women's popular fiction within her writing. Her muted discourse resists and subverts those cultural conventions that silence any mention of the expected outcome of a woman's role as wife—pregnancy—in order to fulfill the sacred role of motherhood.

Chopin first openly writes about pregnancy in her short story "Athenaise," in which the young wife who runs away from her husband returns when she delightedly discovers she is pregnant. Some nineteenth-century critics found the story "coarse," but others were charmed by the happy resolution (Toth 303). Chopin perhaps takes advantage of the latitude allowed by her "local colorist" status to further subvert the tradition in *The Awakening* by calling the pregnant Adele a "sensuous Madonna." Edna, representative of mainstream Protestant America, is "shocked" by the intimate details of pregnancy and childbirth that the Creole women and men discuss so matter of factly. Chopin's contemporary critics, however, furious with Edna's lack of remorse for her adultery and Chopin's lack of censure of Edna's actions, failed to notice the novel's references to a "bountifully pregnant woman, glorying in her condition" (Toth 332).

In addition to the dominant discourse of Adele's pregnancy, however, Chopin at the same time depicts Edna's awakening as a pregnancy through a muted, subversive voice. The first clue to Chopin's possibly deliberate use of the language of pregnancy can be found in the novel's structure of thirty-nine chapters, a number suggestive of an average pregnancy that lasts from thirty-eight to forty-two weeks. Moreover, the events within the chapters correspond to various experiences documented in normal pregnancies. Turning to the text, it seems likely that Edna's conception of her individual self occurs in early summer as the novel opens, in the sea where she has been trying to learn to swim. The sea is both Edna's mother and lover; like a woman, the sea is sexual, sensual, maternal, and erotic. Stone calls the sea "the source of all life" that becomes "the central symbol for Edna's birthing of a new self" (25). Elaine Showalter reminds us that the sea is commonly given feminine attributes and often compared to the female body, which is "prone to wetness, blood, milk, tears, and amniotic fluid" (81). Through the sea's influence a "ponderous weight of wisdom" descends upon Edna's soul, "more wisdom than the Holy Ghost is usually pleased to vouchsafe to any woman" (*Awakening* 57), recalling the annunciation of the Virgin Mary and her conception of Jesus through the power of the Holy Ghost. This figurative evocation of the Virgin is an example of what Margaret Homans calls "bearing the word," a practice by which female writers literalize a female experience such as conception (28-29).

Further subtle pregnancy imagery abounds in Chapter VI, corresponding to Edna's sixth week of pregnancy, a time when many women are only vaguely aware of the changes going on inside them. Perceiving the first stirrings of life that are "beginning to dawn dimly within," Edna starts "to realize her position in the universe as a human being, and to recognize her relations as an individual to the *world within* and about her" (*Awakening* 57 emphasis added). This beginning is "necessarily vague, tangled, chaotic, and exceedingly disturbing" (57), a genuine description of pregnancy. The disturbance is caused by what Rich identifies as "the fear of change, of transformation, of the unfamiliar" (167). Modern pregnancy handbooks agree that there is "something incomprehensible about the beginnings of life. And by becoming pregnant we open ourselves to changes and complications. We become much more aware of being vulnerable" (*Our Bodies* 421). Edna's growing awareness of her place in the universe is the crux of her awakening to her new self.

During pregnancy a woman may feel heightened perceptions and "a feeling of being in love" (*Our Bodies* 418), and the "pregnant" Edna becomes keenly sensitive. In such a receptive condition, other "subtle and apparent" influences on the island begin "to loosen a little the mantle of reserve" Edna has worn for many years (*Awakening* 57). On August 28 her inner condition coalesces. Early in the morning she shares her first intimate experience with a woman, as Adele clasps her hand "firmly and warmly," murmuring endearments. Edna responds, putting her head on Adele's shoulder as she reveals her innermost thoughts candidly for the first time in her life, feeling that bond "which we call sympathy, which we might as well call love" (*Awakening* 58). In the early evening another woman, Mlle. Reisz, touches her by playing the piano with such artistry that Edna's passions are "aroused within her soul," moving her to tremble and choke on her blinding tears. "Unaccustomed to an outward and spoken expression of affection, either in herself or in others" (*Awakening* 61), she then is caressed for the second time that day. Later that evening, in a state of exhilaration, she suddenly overcomes her final inhibitions and begins to swim, imbued with "some power of significant import" with which to "control the working of her body and soul" (72). Finally, she and Robert share moments of silence that are "pregnant with the first-felt throbbings of desire" as her sexual awakening commences (77). Chopin's only use of the word "pregnant" in the novel illustrates what Homans calls a "conspicuous metaphor" that translates a figure "into an actual event or circumstance" (30). Chopin boldly uses this valued, meaningful word to identify covertly her hidden discourse; by calling silence pregnant, pregnancy within the text is no longer silenced.

Chopin subtly links the progression of Edna's awakening and metaphoric pregnancy to Adele's literal pregnancy, drawing on her own intimate knowledge of the emotional and physical manifestations of pregnancy. While Adele thrives in her role as "mother-woman," for Edna, pregnancy is what Rich describes as "the extinguishing of an earlier self," heralding "enormous changes" for the woman (167). Edna is subtly aware of some kind of change within, "that she herself—her present self—was in some way different from the other self," but she does "not yet suspect" the "new conditions in herself" (*Awakening* 88). Both Edna and Adele are easily fatigued, for instance, a common complaint especially in early pregnancy. Pregnant women need more sleep than usual and are urged to nap or rest often because their bodies are undergoing such enormous changes. An early critic, George Arms, is amused by what he asserts is Chopin's consciously allowing "Edna to do an inordinate amount of sleeping throughout the novel, in spite of her underlying vitality" (200); Arms misses the hidden second voice, unable to detect the language of pregnancy. Both women also exhibit other early signs of pregnancy such as faintness, headaches, and dizziness. When Edna goes to church on the *Cheniere Caminada* with Robert, for example, her head aches, the lights seem to sway, and she feels faint. Adele also complains of faintness one afternoon, to which Edna responds by bathing her face and fanning her. Edna suspects, however, that Adele is merely looking for attention because "the rose tint had never faded from her friend's face" (*Awakening* 56).

Chopin clearly observes the details of women's lives as she contrasts various experiences during pregnancy. Edna and Adele exhibit opposite—but normal—behaviors concerning food, for instance. Subscribing to the popular medical philosophy of the late nineteenth century that pregnancy is an illness and a woman is what Dr. Mandelet calls a "very peculiar and delicate organism" (*Awakening* 119), Adele is most particular about what she eats; Edna's appetite, on the other hand, is lusty and continues to grow. The 1896 medical advice book *Glory of Woman* notes that some pregnant women have "wretched appetites; they regularly loathe their food and dread the approach of meal-times. Other women, in contrast, eat more heartily during pregnancy than any other period of their lives—they are absolutely ravenous, and can scarcely satisfy their hunger" (Allen 112). Edna represents such women, to whom "everything edible looks, tastes, smells, even feels good" (Gillespie 67). For example, Robert delightedly prepares a hearty meal for Edna, "childishly gratified to discover her appetite, and to see the relish with which she ate the food" (*Awakening* 86). Contrast this robust meal to the earlier scene in which he solicitously serves Adele a dainty cup of bouillon and a "flaky cracker or two" (66). Near the end of their respective pregnancies, Adele declines the invitation to Edna's birthday party because she is ill and "unpresentable" (153). Thanking Edna for the delicious food gifts from the party, she moans that she "has so little appetite" (153). Edna, meanwhile, continues to enjoy large meals, alcohol, and coffee, both alone and with company.

Another difference in the two pregnancies is the approach to exercise. While Adele subscribes to the maxim of her time to avoid vigorous exercise, Edna is well ahead of her contemporaries. In the 1890s a woman was cautioned that as soon as she has "the slightest suspicion that she is *enceinte,* she must be careful in the taking of exercise" (Allen 115), and Adele stays home all day "except to take a languid walk around the block with her husband after nightfall" (*Awakening* 130). Modern pregnancy handbooks, on the other hand, promote physical activity and brisk exercise to foster a general feeling of well being, and Edna enjoys long walks. She feels "so sorry for women who don't like to walk; they miss so much—so many rare little glimpses of life; and we women learn so little of life on the whole" (*Awakening* 165). Similarly, Adele claims she cannot dance because of her "condition," while Edna whirls through five dances, enjoying herself. It is not clear whether Adele ever swims, but perhaps she does not because "sea-bathing" was not recommended for pregnant women in the nineteenth century, although a "change of air to the coast (provided it be not too far away from home), and inhaling the sea-breezes, may brace her, and ward off the tendency" to miscarry (Allen 115). Edna, on the other hand, "intoxicated with her newly conquered power" (*Awakening* 74) over the sea, spends much of her time in the water because swimming gives her such pleasure, reinforcing the image of herself as a gestating fetus in the amniotic fluid.

In her open, expectant state, Edna experiences sensations commonly reported by many pregnant women in the late twentieth century, including feelings of being fertile, potent, or creative (*Our Bodies* 418). While Adele keeps her "mother-woman" hands busy sewing winter baby clothes, Edna devotes herself to painting, a non-domestic pursuit. Unlike Adele, whose piano was undoubtedly a part of the family's living area, Edna insists on creating a room of her own, "a bright room in the top of the house" in which to paint (*Awakening* 108). Her "gravid" state impels her toward an assertiveness as she leaves behind her former submissive self.

We do not find out much else about Adele from the brief glimpses we are given until she goes into labor, in keeping with nineteenth-century Victorian attitudes; proper women confined themselves during pregnancy to avoid confronting polite society with the evidence of their sexual activity. While Chopin allows Adele to hide, however, she continues to describe Edna's activities with the language of pregnancy. For instance, Edna is often moved "to dreams, to thoughtfulness" and to tears (*Awakening* 57), matching descriptions in modern pregnancy manuals of moodiness or "emotional lability" as well as vivid dreams experienced by all pregnant women at one time or another (*Our Bodies* 421). In Chapter XX, for example, corresponding to her second trimester,

Edna discovers "many a sunny, sleepy corner, fashioned to dream in," finding it "good to dream" (*Awakening* 109). Dreams in pregnancy relay messages and information about the self that a woman would not usually have access to (Hotchner 231); when Edna dreams of Mrs. Highcamp telling Arobin that "so much talent has been neglected" (*Awakening* 129), Edna's growing inner self recognizes the societal restrictions placed on her talents. Clearly Chopin has a message for women: the heightened perceptions and sensuous nature of pregnancy are healthy and natural and should be enjoyed.

One sure sign of pregnancy is the quickening, when a woman first feels the movements of the fetus; it usually occurs between the eighteenth and twentieth weeks, in the second trimester. Pregnancy handbooks, both modern and historic, describe this feeling of quickening as an unexpected fluttering, bumping or leaping sensation which is gentle and of short duration, and note that many women liken it to the "fluttering of a bird" (Allen 109). Edna's quickening occurs at the end of Chapter XVIII, corresponding to the eighteenth week of pregnancy, as Edna reflects on the domestic life that Adele leads. Unexpectedly, the "unsought, extraneous impression" of the descriptive phrase "life's delirium" flashes through her thoughts; this flashing sensation could be the kicking of her growing inner self that protests Adele's "colorless existence which never uplifted its possessor beyond the region of blind contentment" (*Awakening* 107). This sensation could symbolize what literary critic Martha Fodaski Black calls the "yearning for new life [that] quickens in Edna" (102). While Chopin may not have deliberately inserted this allusion to quickening in the text, she is undoubtedly familiar with the sensation from her own six pregnancies.

Chopin frequently alludes to the outward signs of Edna's "pregnancy" as Edna enters her second trimester, a time when a woman "feels good, fulfilled, and quite benign about the vicissitudes of the world around her. The attractiveness of a clear complexion, bright eyes, facial expressions of alert intelligence, and a congruent posture are recognized and appreciated socially" (Rubin 65). Even early in Edna's gestation her eyes are "quick and bright" (*Awakening* 45) and "bright and wide awake" (85). Her metaphoric "condition" causes people to comment on her good looks. Madame Lebrun tells Victor "how handsome" Edna looks. Victor agrees, calling her "Ravishing! . . . Some way she doesn't seem like the same woman" (113). That same afternoon Mlle. Reisz compliments Edna, "Always handsome! always healthy! always contented!" (114). Later at dinner the doctor observes Edna, noting "a subtle change which had transformed her from the listless woman he had known into a being who, for the moment, seemed palpitant with the forces of life. . . . She reminded him of some beautiful, sleek animal waking up in the sun" (123). A worried Leonce, however, thinks Edna is "not herself," but he fails to see that she is actually "becoming herself" (*Awakening* 108); pregnancy causes a woman to be "transformed" right before everyone's eyes (Hotchner 255). One distinct advantage of Edna's metaphoric pregnancy, of course, is that she does not gain weight, although at the beginning of her third trimester, the narrator remarks that Edna's chin is "growing a little full and double" (*Awakening* 138). While she does not display an enlarging belly, she does experience the typical shifting center of gravity, feeling off-balance and uncomfortable as with a literal pregnancy and viewing her formerly secure environment as "an alien world" (*Awakening* 104).

In Chapter XXVII, as Edna enters the final trimester of her metaphoric pregnancy, she turns inward, concentrating on the new person she is becoming to "determine what character of a woman" she is, as she tells Arobin (138). Modern pregnancy handbooks describe pregnancy as a "life crisis" in which a woman gains new insights and outlooks because everything is changing. Edna begins to see her life with new eyes, perhaps because pregnancy is, as Rich declares, "one way of knowing and coming to terms with our bodies, of discovering our physical and psychic resources" (157). Although a pregnant woman feels the new life inside her, this living presence is a tangible experience to her that does not become real to other people until after the baby is born.

A few weeks before delivery a woman also begins to experience a genuine fear and dread of death, for herself and the baby. In order to occupy their minds from worrying about the impending labor, many women experience an outburst of energy in which they clean, cook and organize so that their houses are in "dying order or ready for a very welcome arrival" (Rubin 47). This energy signals what is often called the "nesting" phase as labor approaches. Edna enters the nesting phase when she decides to move to her own "pigeon house," evoking bird imagery again as she creates her own nursery/nest. Gripped by "a feverish anxiety" (*Awakening* 139), she hastens her preparations for the move, cleaning and packing in order to occupy her new home within two days. This sense of time running out is common in late pregnancy as women urgently prepare for birth, and Chopin surely draws from her own experience for this scene.

Pregnancy is a natural process with its own cycles; one of the last cycles is labor, which "has its own unique rhythm with periods of intense activity, plateau periods and rest periods" (*Our Bodies* 440). Once Adele goes into labor, she sends for Edna, who leaves Robert immediately just as it seems likely they will consummate their relationship. Although Adele had shocked Edna at Grand Isle by telling Monsieur Farival all the intimate details of her accouchements, the message she sends to Edna is that she has "been taken sick," again reinforcing the late nineteenth-century notion of pregnancy as pathology rather than natural process (*Awakening* 167). When Edna arrives for Adele's "hour of trial" (153), she finds her friend in what Ivy Schweitzer perceptively describes as transition, the tempestuous first stage of labor (180). Adele no longer looks like the ideal woman, with her face "drawn and pinched, her sweet blue eyes haggard and unnatural," pacing uncontrollably and babbling hysterically (*Awakening* 169). Because Edna does not remember her own deliveries and, unlike the Creoles, never discusses these private matters with anyone, her naivete leaves her unprepared for the "scene of torture" that she witnesses during Adele's delivery. Afterward, her romantic illusions about motherhood disappear in a "flaming, outspoken revolt against the ways of Nature" (*Awakening* 170).

Meanwhile, throughout Adele's labor, Edna has been in labor herself. During Adele's contractions Edna starts to "feel uneasy" and is "seized with a vague dread" (*Awakening* 170), echoing earlier references to the imminent danger of childbirth. Still stunned from Adele's delivery, Edna begins her own transition phase, "voicing the incoherency of her thoughts" to Dr. Mandelet, who cannot help her (171). Arriving home, Edna anticipates her reunion with Robert, growing "numb with the intoxication of expectancy" (172), phrasing that deliberately invokes the experience of anesthesia during labor. Reaching a plateau in her labor, and devastated by Robert's betrayal, she spends a long, sleepless night thinking about many things, including her children.

The final chapter corresponds to the beginning of week thirty-nine of Edna's pregnancy. Refusing to be confined to her house and then bedroom during labor as Adele was, Edna instinctively journeys to Grand Isle to be with her natural mother/lover, thus breaking out of the literal domestic confinement that circumscribed the lives of nineteenth-century women. Now in the final stage of labor, she takes off her bathing suit, standing naked for the first time without the "unpleasant, pricking" conventions of society, which Dr. Mandelet has correctly identified as "arbitrary conditions which we create, and which we feel obliged to maintain at any cost" (*Awakening* 171). A naked Edna feels "strange" and "delicious," "like some new-born creature" (175). To many modern critics, these words signal Edna's rebirth. Chopin's maternal subtext, however, helps us realize that Edna has not yet given birth to herself. While Adele had attendants at her delivery, Edna has only her mother, the sea, with its sensuous touch and soft embrace. Entering the water naked, Edna prepares to give birth in a manner advocated by progressive twentieth-century birthing specialists. She deliberately swims with a "long, sweeping stroke" (176); her rhythmic, contraction-like strokes continue until her arms and legs grow tired. During this final phase of labor women often "want to just rest" (*Our Bodies* 445). Edna needs to rest from the exhaustion "pressing upon and overpowering her" and "the old terror" of death that "flames up for just an instant and then recedes" (*Awakening* 176). This is the same terror she felt when she first learned to swim, underscoring the life and death implicit in childbirth.

Edna's labor is told from her point of view, again illustrating Chopin's intimate familiarity as participant in this woman-centered event. Modern childbirth literature corroborates the laboring woman's experience: "The eyes are usually closed and when open are unseeing, so that there is little or no visual stimulation, only tactile and sound conduction. Soft, rhythmical sounds, coming from outside self, seem to provide an 'outside' for the self, a containment by surrounding" (Rubin 74). The sea contains Edna, embracing her; each memory rolls over her like a contraction. Edna, like Adele, is physically exhausted; unlike the "scene of torture" of Adele's labor, however, the final images of the novel are uplifting, not defeating. Instead of the heavy odor of chloroform of her previous deliveries, Edna now smells flowers (Schweitzer 186). She also hears the hum of bees, underscoring the fecundity of nature that has been woven throughout the story.

The language of the final scene invokes Edna's "delivery," which leads us to ask, delivery from what, and to what? As Edna "delivers" her new self, the dominant discourse suggests drowning, allowing readers to think that Edna has chosen suicide to escape from her children or to kill her new-born self because there is no place in the world for it. Chopin subverts this conventional nineteenth-century punishment, however, by describing Edna's implied death in pleasant terms. Instead of creating a scene reminiscent of Emma Bovary's famous and horribly painful death, Chopin depicts what Sandra Gilbert calls an "ambiguously triumphant awakening" (33) that raises but does not answer questions. The circular nature of the novel allows for both death and rebirth, presaging a new beginning in the new century; the ambiguity highlights the lack of role models available for women. If there is a new creature, what happens next? How will this creature survive?

No immediate answer is offered, but the novel's rediscovery some seventy years later ironically provides new life for the text. Continued critical attention proves Wolff's assertion that Chopin "had invented a powerful (and thus threatening) discourse for feminine sexuality" in her novel ("Un-Utterable" 18). Such discourse had to be suppressed at the turn of the last century, but it has resurfaced, demanding recognition now that pregnancy and childbirth have become controllable events and are beginning to be subjects worthy of literary attention. Chopin's brilliant use of the language of pregnancy for both a literal and metaphoric life-changing event underscores the centrality and universality of this natural process for women, and anticipates questions asked by modern critics. Spender, for example, compares the literary value of the male experience of war with the female experience of childbirth, noting that before a battle, many men believe they are risking death. She asks where the literature is that gives voice to the millions of women who "on the eve of giving birth have faced the very same fate?" (115). Chopin, one of the first writers to boldly resist the conventions surrounding pregnancy and childbirth, subtly writes in and subverts the dominant discourse to provide both the language and a way to discuss such silenced but universal concerns.

Acknowledgments

I wish to thank Barbara Murray and Kathryn Seidel for their insightful comments. Portions of this essay were read at the 1996 Twentieth-Century Literature Conference in Louisville and the 1996 M/MLA Conference in Minneapolis.

Works Cited

Allen, Monfort B., M.D., and Amelia C. McGregor, M.D. *The Glory of Woman, or Love, Marriage and Maternity*. Chicago: American Publishing House, 1896.

Arms, George. "Contrasting Forces in the Novel." Kate Chopin. *The Awakening*. Margo Culley. 2nd ed. New York: Norton, 1994. 198-202.

Black, Martha Fodaski. "The Quintessence of Chopinism." *Kate Chopin Reconsidered: Beyond the Bayou*. Ed. Lynda S. Boren and Sara deSaussure Davis. Baton Rouge: Louisiana State UP, 1992. 95-113.

Chopin, Kate. *The Awakening and Selected Stories*. Ed. Sandra M. Gilbert. New York: Penguin, 1983.

Gilbert, Sandra M. "The Second Coming of Aphrodite." Kate Chopin. *The Awakening and Selected Stories*. Ed. Sandra M. Gilbert. New York: Penguin, 1983. 7-33.

Gillespie, Clark, M.D. *Your Pregnancy Month by Month*. New York: Harper & Row, 1985.

Homans, Margaret. *Bearing the Word*. Chicago: U of Chicago P, 1986.

Hotchner, Tracy. *Pregnancy and Childbirth*. New York: Avon Books, 1990.

Jacobsen, Cheryl L. Rose. "Dr. Mandelet's Real Life Counterparts and Their Advice Books: Setting a Context for Edna's Revolt." *Perspectives on Kate Chopin*. Ed. Grady Ballenger, et al. Natchitoches, LA: Northwestern State UP, 1990. 101-25.

The New Our Bodies, Ourselves. The Boston Women's Health Book Collective. 2nd ed. New York: Touchstone, 1992.

Rich, Adrienne. *Of Woman Born: Motherhood as Experience and Institution*. Tenth anniversary ed. New York: Norton, 1986.

Riley, Madeleine. *Brought to Bed*. New York: A. S. Barnes, 1968.

Rubin, Reva. *Maternal Identity and the Maternal Experience*. New York: Springer, 1984.

Schor, Naomi. "Feminist and Gender Studies." *Introduction to Scholarship in Modern Languages and Literatures*. 2nd ed. Ed. Joseph Gibaldi. New York: The Modern Language Association of America, 1992. 262-87.

Schweitzer, Ivy. "Maternal Discourse and the Romance of Self-Possession in Kate Chopin's *The Awakening*." *Boundary* 17 (1990): 158-86.

Seyersted, Per. *Kate Chopin: A Critical Biography*. Baton Rouge: Louisiana State UP, 1969.

Showalter, Elaine. *Sister's Choice*. Oxford: Clarendon P, 1991.

Skaggs, Peggy. *Kate Chopin*. Boston: Twayne, 1985.

Spender, Dale. *The Writing or the Sex?* New York: Pergamon P, 1989.

Stone, Carole. "The Female Artist in Kate Chopin's *The Awakening*: Birth and Creativity." *Women's Studies* 13 (1986): 23-32.

Thomas, Heather Kirk. "Kate Chopin's Scribbling Women and the American Literary Marketplace." *Studies in American Fiction* 23.1 (1995): 19-34.

Toth, Emily. *Kate Chopin*. New York: William Morrow, 1990.

Wolff, Cynthia Griffin. "Thanatos and Eros: Kate Chopin's *The Awakening*." *Kate Chopin. The Awakening*. Ed. Nancy A. Walker. Boston: Bedford, 1993. 233-58.

——. "Un-Utterable Longing: The Discourse of Feminine Sexuality in *The Awakening*." *Studies in American Fiction* 24.1 (1996): 3-22.

5

SOUTHERN CONCEPTIONS:

FEMINIST PROCREATION IN JULIA PETERKIN'S

SCARLET SISTER MARY AND FRANCES NEWMAN'S

THE HARD-BOILED VIRGIN

Debra Beilke

While recent decades have spawned a proliferation of feminist scholarship on pregnancy, childbirth, and maternal subjectivity, important lacunae still remain.[1] E. Ann Kaplan, for example, argues that theoretical difficulties arise from the intellectual isolation between different modes of inquiry into maternal experience, such as the psychoanalytic and the sociological (217). Alice Adams makes a similar point when she asserts that most representations of motherhood are considered *either* from an emotional/biological *or* from a social/economic perspective (423). Studying the novels of two white southern women writers of the 1920s, Julia Peterkin's *Scarlet Sister Mary* (1928) and Frances Newman's *The Hard-Boiled Virgin* (1926), can help us move beyond this impasse by illuminating the complex interactions between the social and the psychological registers in the construction of maternal subjectivity. These two novels can be fruitfully read alongside Lillian Smith's *Killers of the Dream* and W. J. Cash's *Mind of the South,* classic explorations of the southern psyche, as insightful ruminations on the psychological and erotic side-effects—the "strange fruit"—of the rigid race, class, and gender inequalities of the pre-Civil Rights South.

In writing their novels, both Peterkin and Newman grappled with the complex and anxious question of how motherhood forms or deforms female identity in the 1920s, this post-suffrage, putatively "liberated" era for women. Because, however, racial issues were at the forefront of Peterkin's mind, while upper-class concerns were central for Newman, the two authors provide diametrically opposed viewpoints of the role of maternity in constructing a vision of female identity unhampered by sexism. Julia Peterkin's primitivist representation of a black heroine in *Scarlet Sister Mary* propels her vision of childbirth and midwifery as a means of accessing women's natural powers of the body, an embodied vitality which leads to greater equality between the sexes. On the other hand, Frances Newman's acute sensitivity to upper-class manners greatly intensifies her protagonist's fear of pregnancy and childbirth in *The Hard-Boiled Virgin*. Recognizing that the exigencies of upper class southern manners harshly repress women's bodies and minds, her heroine refuses to participate in the reproduction of this system. Despite their differences, however, both texts highlight the complex interaction between the psychological and social registers in representing maternal subjectivity. Although her utopian vision of maternal subjectivity relies for its effect on naturalist imagery, Peterkin's imagination is in fact profoundly mediated by the social realm, more specifically the racism of her southern plantation society. And while the supposedly neurotic behavior of "hard-boiled virgin" Katharine Faraday has often been viewed by critics as an individual, psychological problem, her rejection of marriage and procreation is in fact a political reaction to social injustice.

The debate over the relationship between sexuality, maternity, and female identity evinced in these texts can be better understood in light of the social convulsions in the United States of the 1920s. On the one hand, the 1920s witnessed dramatic changes in the mainstream culture's expectations of female sexuality. This new sexual order, according to Emilio and Freedman, redefined womanhood to include (heterosexual) eroticism (233). Whereas acceptable sexuality for white middle-class women had previously been synonymous with marital reproduction, this new era emphasized the individualistic pursuit of sexual pleasure for both men and women.

But while mainstream culture sanctioned a greater degree of public heterosexual assertion, at the same time the rise of the male experts in childbirth and child rearing functioned to *diminish* women's traditional authority in this realm. Mothers, according to Dorothy Brown, were coming under increasing control and surveillance of the experts, with their previously sacrosanct domain now being invaded by scientific scrutiny (117). This invasion of the male experts stemmed, according to Barbara Ehrenreich and Deirdre English, from the masculinist imagination's recent "discovery" of the child as "the leading figure in the family," a "kind of evolutionary protoplasm" (191). Now that they recognized the importance of child-rearing, the experts deemed the job too important to be left in the sole hands of women, whether in the North or the South. Male scientific expertise was considered not only superior but also necessary in order to save children from the dangers of ignorant mothers. Unfortunately, rather than offering any material help in child-rearing tasks, the experts instead offered only advice, warnings, and instructions. In so doing, they not only insulted women's traditional childcare knowledge, but also subjected many mothers to increased feelings of inadequacy, guilt, and anxiety. As Ann Firor Scott observes: "In the past when children turned out badly, it could be seen as the will of God or the working out of inherent human nature; now it could be attributed to the failure of the mother to know enough or practice enough of what she knew" (220-21). The male experts, then, tried and often succeeded in undermining women's confidence in their child rearing abilities. As Ehrenreich and English aptly phrase it, "When the experts enter the area of child raising, they step into what had been, for better or worse, the irreducible core of women's existence, the last refuge of her skills and dignity" (191).

This combination of increased expectations for women to achieve sexual pleasure in conjunction with decreased confidence in their abilities to nurture their offspring led, not surprisingly, to anxiety and confusion over the parameters of female identity for American women of the 1920s. Both Julia Peterkin and Frances Newman respond to this cultural climate in a spirit of feminist resistance, although their individual brands of resistance vary dramatically, and are undergirded by their specific social positions and concerns. Peterkin resists the onslaught against women's realm of expertise by emphasizing women's natural strength and wisdom in the reproductive arena, while Newman's protagonist resists by retreating from the sexual marketplace altogether, creating instead a theory of superior virginal aesthetics.

Julia Peterkin's Scarlet Sister Mary

Julia Peterkin's portrayal of female identity as empowered through childbirth must be understood within the context of her position as a plantation owner in the segregated South. From 1903, when she married a planter, to her death in 1961, Julia Peterkin was the white mistress of a large (2,000-acre) and isolated cotton plantation near Fort Motte, South Carolina. (Although slavery had long since been abolished by this time, the material conditions of Peterkin and her laborers mirrored those of the antebellum period.) Fascinated with the lives of her 500 black employees, she wrote several acclaimed books of fiction devoted exclusively to their folkways.

Scarlet Sister Mary, which sold over a million copies and garnered a Pulitzer Prize for its author in 1929, recounts the story of Mary Pinesett, an African American plantation laborer considered "scarlet" because of her premarital pregnancy and numerous post-marital lovers. At a very young age, Mary falls deeply in love with, becomes impregnated by, and marries a handsome but domineering man named July.

Their marriage soon disintegrates, however, when July bullies and neglects Mary and finally runs away with another woman. After a period of depression, Mary rises from the ashes of despondency and becomes strong and happy again, henceforth using men only for physical pleasure. Part of the reason for her renewed vitality is her fecundity: Mary bears nine children by several different fathers. Her births are amazingly easy—almost painless—and rather than leading to victimization or exhaustion, her fertility contributes to her exuberant vitality. Although the church-going members of the plantation quarters frown upon Mary's lifestyle, she is not ostracized, and finds her life generally satisfactory.

Certain biographical information about Peterkin is necessary to understand the significance of her portrayal of easy fecundity. Despite Peterkin's racial privilege, she still lacked control over her own reproductive capacities because of her gender. According to historian Elizabeth Robeson, after the birth in 1904 of Peterkin's only child, her father, Dr. Mood, performed a tubal ligation on her. As Robeson puts it, "On a plantation filled with midwives, Dr. Mood delivered his daughter's baby and following the birth declared her unfit to bear any more children. While Julia Peterkin lay unconscious, Dr. Mood secured the consent of her husband to sterilize her" (769). Robeson asserts that the reasons for the sterilization are "elusive," but the fact that the procedure was performed without her consent "embittered Julia Peterkin for the rest of her life" (769).

Given this biographical information about the author, her novel's primitivist romanticization of black women's "natural" powers of the body can be read as a feminist critique of white patriarchal, scientific "progress." In other words, while Peterkin has usually been read as a realistic, "local color" writer, I think *Scarlet Sister Mary* is more fruitfully read as feminist primitivist fantasy. Using insights gained from Marianna Torgovnick's *Gone Primitive,* I contend that the African Americans Peterkin represent serve as "grist" for her "fantasy mill" (153), allowing her obliquely to voice desires, dreams, and social criticism that would otherwise have been forbidden to a respectable southern lady. As Toni Morrison argues, "Just as entertainers, through or by association with blackface, could render permissible topics that otherwise would have been taboo, so American writers were able to employ an imagined Africanist person to articulate and imaginatively act out the forbidden in American culture" (66). Peterkin creates the fictional character of Scarlet Sister Mary in order to articulate "forbidden" critiques of patriarchal control over women's bodies, including their reproductive capacities.

In an uncomfortable blend of racism and feminism, Peterkin employs primitivist tropes of black women's supposed closeness to nature in order to imagine an independent woman whose "natural" lifestyle accesses the powers of the maternal body. This same strategy also enables Peterkin to represent midwifery as a site of female wisdom superior to that of the male scientific "experts." The "natural" fecundity and resistance to patriarchal authority of her heroine Mary stands in stark contrast to the "unnatural" barrenness and submission Peterkin herself was forced to endure in her involuntary sterilization.

In keeping with modernist primitivist tropes, the text discursively allies the plantation laborers in general and Mary in particular with nature. Isolated from the larger society, Peterkin depicts the Blue Brook plantation culture as natural and simplistic, unsullied by contact with modernity: "The lack of roads and bridges afforded them little contact with the outside world, and so, instead of going away to seek new fortunes, new advantages, easier work and more money, they kept faithful to the old life, contented with old ways and beliefs, holding fast to old traditions and superstitions" (10). Mary, however, "like a garden where flowers blossom the whole year through" (175), is even more "natural" than most, since she rejects the "civilizing" forces of Christianity that most of the plantation dwellers embrace. Compared to a "weed" (12), a "cat" (26), a "grey fox" (32), a "bird" (18) and a "flower" (18) among other things, she has never been more than five miles from home and is deeply connected to the land: "The very earth here was part of herself, and it held her so fast she could never leave it, no matter what came" (107).

Mary's close connection to nature is intricately related to her abundant fertility and childbearing ease. Underscoring the naturalness of her heroine's fertility, Peterkin juxtaposes the birth of Mary's first child with a long, lyrical description of nature in bloom. Like Mary, "the whole earth was full of birthing and growing" (58). Such descriptions suggest that childbirth is not a disease to be treated by medical experts or a shameful event which needs to be "confined," but a natural source of vitality and power. The plantation folk, for example, recognize the power of pregnant women in their rituals:

A woman who is about to bear a child has a strangely good hand for planting seed; something magic in her touch makes the seed sprout quickly and grow fast and mature in half the regular time. Everybody in the Quarters who planted a winter vegetable garden wanted Mary to drop the seed. [Furthermore,] [m]edicines brewed by a woman at such a time have more strength to cure ailments. (51)

Within the setting of the Blue Brook plantation, then, pregnancy as Peterkin describes it is a joyful testimony to the natural powers of the female body.

Peterkin emphasizes the power and strength of the female body by portraying Mary as almost immune to pain, even in labor. This tribute to the powers of the black female body, unfortunately, has a disturbing side in that it sustains racist stereotypes that women of color feel less pain than white women. Nineteenth- and early twentieth-century Americans commonly believed that certain groups of people felt more pain than others. Although women were supposed to be more sensitive to pain than men, lower-class women and women of color were perceived to feel less pain than middle and upper-class white women. Martin Pernick, for example, documents the belief by southern whites that "Negro mothers 'were not subject to the . . . pain which attended women of the better classes in giving birth'" (156). Peterkin seems to accept this racist belief because she represents Mary as so robust that physical pain is almost unknown to her, whether in the labor of childbirth or the labor of picking cotton. More than once the narrator reminds us that, for Mary, "birthing children was not so bad. It was as easy for her as to pop her fingers" (203). Labor, the novel suggests, is so easy for her because she is animal-like in her physicality, bearing her offspring quietly and without complaint:

Mary had a brave heart. She had done well in her first trial at birthing a child. A woman with plenty of experience could have done no better. *God must have blessed her with the same wisdom he gave to the beasts,* who know well when the time comes to birth their young, and instead of complaining of God's ways, as people do, go off alone without a word, and struggle with their labor as best they can. (61, emphasis added)

Although Mary does in fact feel "a spasm of pain" (60), her animal-like naturalness enables her to bear it stoically, rather than make a huge fuss like so many women do. Mary's ease in giving birth is matched by her ease in raising her children. They practically raise themselves, to no apparent harm.

Although Peterkin has often been praised for her objective realism, her depiction of Mary's childbearing and child rearing experiences seems clearly situated in the realm of fantasy.[2] Documenting the realities of African American women's lives during this historical period, Jacqueline Jones refutes Peterkin's primitivist vision of black women's robust fertility and unbreakable strength; she reports that the combination of hard physical labor, poverty and repeated childbirth resulted, not surprisingly, in poor health and a decline in fertility rates for black women.

Peterkin, however, is less interested in realism than in imagining the pleasures of the female body outside a dominant male economy in which women are merely objects of male exchange. From a feminist point of view, one of the advantages of Peterkin's primitivism is that it allows her to portray Mary as a sexual *subject,* not a helpless object of male lust. She has numerous short-term lovers by choice, not because she can't "keep a man." After her first heartbreak, she realizes that "men are the queerest of all God's creatures. Poor fools, not one of them worth a headache, or a teardrop, and yet, worthless as they are, by means of them her own life had become full and her heart had grown warm and glad again" (178-79). This full life and heart come not from romantic love, but from the sexual pleasure and children men can give her. But because Mary's desires are consistently portrayed as "natural," the reader cannot condemn her actions; therefore, Peterkin's primitivism allows her to resist the sexual double standard.

Mary takes pleasure not only in her sexuality, but also in procreation, finding it physically rejuvenating. For example, after a long struggle with depression because of her husband's desertion, Mary gives birth to her second child, Seraphine, on Christmas Day, suggesting that this child is her "savior." Indeed, the text informs us that after Seraphine's birth, "Mary herself was a new creature. Her heart was light, her eyes sparkled and her laughter rang out as gaily as anybody's . . . sin and Seraphine had agreed with her" (145). Although the Christian women of the plantation quarters age early, Mary remains youthful and attractive throughout her childbearing years, implying that Mary's youthful vitality comes from living according to natural law rather than Christian law. More importantly, however, her "natural" lifestyle also enables her to resist patriarchal oppression. After her husband abandons her and she follows her instincts for pleasure, she becomes much more independent and strong, receiving emotional and material sustenance from her children and her extended family. Peterkin seems to be suggesting that female sexual and social liberation is much more "natural" and beneficial to women than all the artificial restraints required of white southern ladies.

Peterkin also promotes the natural powers of female wisdom in her positive representation of midwifery. Midwife Maum Hannah, Mary's foster mother, is a character who appears in several of Peterkin's works and is always portrayed as a figure of deep wisdom. During the turn of the century period in which *Scarlet Sister Mary* takes place, most babies in the South were brought into the world with the help of (predominantly black) midwives, rather than doctors. Like Peterkin's fictional Maum Hannah, these midwives were highly respected in their rural communities for their dedication and ability. However, the medical establishment of Peterkin's period was engaged in a campaign to eradicate lay midwives in favor of doctor-assisted births, preferably in hospitals. As Barbara Ehrenreich and Deirdre English point out, "Obstetrics-gynecology was America's most rapidly developing specialty, and midwives would just have to get out of the way" (95). This campaign was not only due to the previously discussed invasion of the male experts into the childbirth arena, but also to racial stereotypes of black "grannies" as ignorant, superstitious, and filthy:

As medical professionals worked to define childbirth as a dangerous and potentially pathological event that could not be left to women—especially ignorant immigrant and black midwives—the hospital was promoted as the best place to give birth, and the professional, white male gynecologist was deemed the only appropriate specialist to attend at delivery. (65)

In her portrayal of Maum Hannah, Peterkin attempts to reclaim the power and dignity of midwifery; far from being ignorant, dirty, or dangerous, Maum Hannah is a repository of black female wisdom, a figure revered by everyone. Peterkin further expresses her skepticism of scientific "progress" in the childbirth realm through Mary's laughter. For example, when Maum Hannah is forced by law to go to school to be certified as a midwife,[3] Mary finds it hilarious: "Great Gawd, ain't it de funniest ting you ever did hear?" (166). She goes on to muse on the silliness of white "expertise":

White people are curious things . . . People had come into the world over the same old road ever since Eve birthed Cain and Abel, and now everybody had to learn how to birth children a new way. It was enough to upset the whole world.

White people try to be too smart. If they keep on messing in God's business and trying to change things from the way He meant them to be, the first thing they knew, He would get cross and make Judgment Day wipe the whole world clean of them. (166)

This passage suggests that women's natural realm, which is still being upheld by black midwives, is a site of ancient wisdom dangerous to usurp. Peterkin, then, rejects the new scientific discourses of birth, preferring the naturalistic traditions which afford women more dignity.

In summary, Peterkin's use of feminist primitivism to reclaim the powers of the maternal body and women's natural wisdom exemplifies the complex interplay between the bio-psychological realm of maternal subjectivity and socio-political realm of race relations in the South of the 1920s. Although her strategy contains racist overtones, because she associates black women with nature, she is also able to imagine a world in which women can celebrate the pleasures of the body without any of its attendant pains and uphold the dignity of traditional female knowledge.

Frances Newman's The Hard-Boiled Virgin

Where a primitivist vision of southern black folk culture undergirds Peterkin's conception of maternal subjectivity, Frances Newman's (1883-1928) understanding of upper-class urban southern manners governs her representation of childbirth. Newman's novel *The Hard-Boiled Virgin* (1926) was, like Peterkin's work, widely read in her time, although little known today. This experimental modernist Kunstlerroman tells the story of southern belle Katharine Faraday's coming of age in Atlanta and her double quest to find a husband and to become a writer. Although she succeeds as a writer, Katharine Faraday fails to find a husband or form any satisfying relationships with either men or women. She has many suitors, but her relationships all end quickly; usually she flees as soon as there is any physical contact.

As such, Newman's heroine is very different from Peterkin's Mary; Katharine never marries and never becomes pregnant. She is, nonetheless, obsessed with childbirth, especially its pain, and this fear colors her view of courtship, marriage, gender roles, and southern manners in general. The relationship extends both ways, however; not only does her knowledge of the pain of childbirth color her vision of her society, but her insights into the flaws of upper-class manners at the same time intensifies her fear of reproduction. Because southern manners focus on birth as both a prerequisite for upper-class identity and as an excuse for mandatory female passivity, Katharine rejects her heritage and refuses to marry, becoming instead a "hard-boiled virgin."

One of the major conflicts in this novel centers around two different meanings of the word "birth." When used in the sense of pedigree, "birth" is the definition of a "satisfactory" person: a southern upper-class person is defined as someone with proper lineage, with distinguished ancestors. On the other hand, when used in the sense of "childbirth," the discourse of birth is considered ill-bred because it emphasizes the indelicate realities of the lower body. (In order to avoid confusion, I will henceforth refer to Birth in the sense of pedigree with an upper-case "B," and birth in the sense of childbirth with a lower-case "b.") While in reality high Birth depends directly upon the labor of female bodies, the definition of well-mannered southern ladyhood veils the materiality of the female body. In other words, despite the inevitable connection between the two meanings of the word, a southern lady is supposed to be cognizant of only the "well-mannered" meaning, the sense of distinguished Birth. She should be ignorant of her own bodily functions because "in

Georgia no lady was supposed to know she was a virgin until she had ceased to be one" (174-75).

Katharine Faraday, however, is obsessed with the body, and, although a virgin, is especially haunted by the specter of childbirth. She is painfully sensitive to the fact that while both men and women of the southern upper class are defined by their Birth, women are additionally defined by their ability to give birth, complicating the formation of upper-class female identity. Katharine observes, for example, that "a boy's honourable social situation seemed to be the result of his inability to produce a baby rather than to his ability to produce an idea" (30).

The Hard-Boiled Virgin emphasizes that defining women solely by their ability to give birth sets up a binary of woman as procreative versus man as (intellectually) creative. Such a binary fosters female vapidity and inhibits female intellectual growth. Katharine learns, for example, that if she wants to rouse ardent but honorable passions in young gentlemen, she needs to hide "her more elaborate mental processes" (124) because both boys and grown men "are not usually taken with romantic attachments for little girls who can spell words of five syllables and who can find the eighteenth term of an arithmetical progression" (46). Because the true goal of southern education for girls is to find a husband rather than to develop their minds, Katharine feels fortunate to escape female schooling with her brain intact:

observation showed her that if she had been sent across Peachtree Street to the Misses Rutherford's School, her brain would have been extracted in the process which the Misses Rutherford felt their duty to southern womanhood required, but that the remaining Miss Washington had felt her duty ended when she left the brains of her young ladies in a state of paralysis. (58)

The extraction or, at best, paralysis of female brains is necessary to perpetuate the system in which women are defined as procreators rather than creators. This binary is particularly invidious because, even though women are defined by their bodies, ladies are not allowed to enjoy their bodies, unless they are willing to lose the privileges of upper-class identity.

Newman not only attacks southern manners for its erasure of female intellectual activity, but also because it perpetuates a morally bankrupt upper class through its obsessive love of "good blood." For her, upper-class manners, by which I mean social forms which serve to demarcate one group of people from another, are nothing more than empty markers of a status inherited from one's family. For example, social forms such as membership in the Piedmont Driving Club, dancing at a Cotillion, belonging to Saint Luke's Protestant Episcopal Church, or "giving lunches for girls who were staying with important girls and for girls who lived in important towns" (24) all announce elite identity. While these markers may not mean anything to an outsider, they are all crucial for members of the Atlanta upper crust because they delineate class boundaries. These class boundaries, in turn, originate in having the proper ancestors, such as those whose "great-grandfathers had given their names to the counties of the more distinguished southern states" (57). Someone, on the other hand, "whose fathers had . . . worn policemen's uniforms or presided over their own green-groceries or lived over their own lime-kilns within the tenacious memory of Katharine Faraday's mother" (128) would be considered "unsatisfactory." Newman's ferocious satire makes it clear that morality, achievement, or good manners in the common sense of the term are irrelevant to being a "well-mannered," or "satisfactory" person within this society, and it is for that reason that her heroine has difficulty finding happiness.

These two objects of Newman's attack—morally bankrupt upper-class identity and the repression of active female desires (be they physical or intellectual)—dovetail in her repeated invocations of the two meanings of the word "birth." If Katharine wants to maintain her privileged class identity, which is based on Birth, she needs to marry a "satisfactory" man—one who is also of high Birth—and give birth to his offspring. Because of this inevitable association between upper-class identity and childbirth, Katharine is terrified of marrying. For her, childbirth is not a glorious event, but one associated mainly with shrieks of pain. Observing the grand spectacle of Sarah Rutledge's wedding, for example, "she was wondering if Sarah Rutledge could be thinking of anything except the dreadful sounds which had come through the opening and closing door of Mrs. Pinckney Rutledge's room on the night before Harriet Rutledge was born" (121). Not only does Katharine immediately associate weddings with coitus and childbirth, but she views this relationship with horror, referring to having babies as a "calamity" (123). This fear of marriage and childbirth simultaneously signifies Katharine's reluctance to reproduce the unearned privileges of Birth and her recognition of women's lack of control over their own bodies and their own fates suggested by birth.

Katharine's reluctance to give up control leads, in turn, to her difficulty "catching" a husband; her failure in the upper-class marriage market stem from her unwillingness to submit to the passivity necessary for a "true" woman. She frequently agonizes over the dating process because she is utterly at the mercy of male desire; she wonders at one point, for example, "why men can ask girls to dance with them and to marry them, and if it is because girls can have babies and men cannot" (93), again underscoring the connection between childbirth and lack of control. And when Katharine finally loses her virginity, she is terrified because she fears she may be pregnant and is "suffering because she did not know what was happening in her own body, and because she could not control her own body" (274). Waiting passively for her period to arrive or not arrive—the "submissive endurance of suspense"—is unbearable to her because "with the one exception of the verb murder, she would rather be the subject of any verb rather than its passive object" (155). (Paradoxically, although Katharine does have sexual intercourse once, she finds that the experience only confirms that she is, in her own words, "hopelessly virginal" [284].) The passivity of women's role in the marriage market as well as the lack of control women experience during pregnancy and childbirth is a major source of Katharine's "frigidity" and her alienation from society.

Katharine, then, avoids marriage because she sees procreation, the inevitable result, as paradigmatic of women's lack of control over their lives. The desire for control explains her increasing interest in virginity, especially its relationship to literary productivity. Although some of Katharine's suitors attempt to persuade her to lose her virginity (with them, of course) in order to improve her writing style, her continued virginity, and her published work adumbrate a counter-argument, a theory of immaculate literary conception. Katharine's published works all hinge upon the theme of virginity. Her first published essay, entitled "Virginal Succession," attempts to prove that sexual activity is bad for a woman's writing style. In it, she argues that "marriage has a bad effect on a woman's writing, and that George Eliot and George Sand might easily have been writing to prove that living in sin is just as injurious to feminine literary style as a union preceded by a civil and a religious ceremony" (235). Furthermore, *The Hard-Boiled Virgin* ends with the successful production and critical admiration of her play "No Sheets," which is about "a girl who could not face the idea of marriage or even of seduction" (257). It seems, then, that Katharine associates writing with "immaculate conception" and prefers such virginal creativity to the pain and lack of control associated with sexual activity. In giving virginal birth to virginal texts, she tries to escape the horrors of the female body by retaining control over it. But, because she is unable to disrupt the binary which views creativity as male and procreativity as female, her success as a writer comes, in her mind, at the cost of her body—which, to her, is the marker of her femininity.

Unfortunately for Katharine, the only way she can write her own life is to reject the female body. She learns while growing up to associate intellectual generativity with the rupture of the female body, a vision that is portrayed most vividly in the following quotation, which takes place when she is an adolescent in the bathtub:

Between her flat chest and her thin legs, she noticed a line she had never noticed before—a delicate line which was slightly browner than the area she thought was her stomach and which began just below the curious little dent her mammy called a navel. And she had a sudden revelation that when her first child . . . came into the world, the part of herself which she thought was her stomach would burst along the delicate brown line, and that she would naturally shriek, and that her daughter would dart into the world like Pallas Athena darting from the brain of Zeus, and that a doctor would then give her ether and sew her up. (36)

This quotation ties together several themes of the novel. First, the discovery of her maturing body and sexuality is shot through with violent visions of childbirth. Also interesting is that she metaphorically envisions giving birth to the goddess of wisdom, suggesting she is able to generate ideas. However, the price of this birth is the literal rupture of the female body. This terrifying vision, then, suggests that in her imagination, Katharine is able to escape her upbringing to the extent that she can envision female intellectual creativity. However, she can escape only partially; unable to deconstruct the binary of female procreativity/male creativity, she feels literary creativity can only come at the price of her ruptured and damaged female body. Perhaps this explains why the novel ends on a note of despair, despite Katharine's success as a writer. She is unable to escape the deeply ingrained ideology that a girl is a "human being who probably could have a baby" and a boy is "one of those favoured beings who are not created to produce babies" (45). Therefore, her success in the world of the mind "proves" to her that she is not a woman.

Images of birth in the *The Hard-Boiled Virgin,* then, occur repeatedly in two separate but intertwined strands of the narrative. One motif represents birth as a signifier for women's enforced passivity and the other invokes birth as the reproduction of unearned upper-class privileges. For an upper-class southern woman character such as Katharine Faraday, the two strands cannot be disentangled: to maintain her class status, she must prove her "femininity" and vice versa. In rejecting childbirth, Katharine simultaneously rejects her privileged class position in southern society.

In summary, despite these two novelists' dramatically different views on procreation, Peterkin and Newman both represent childbirth and pregnancy in ways that resist patriarchal control over women's bodies. Peterkin's primitivist imagination, while racist, allows her to imagine a utopian space where women are magically freed of childbirth pain and emotional dependence on men. Newman's heroine, on the other hand, rejects motherhood and heterosexuality altogether in favor of a feminist, virginal aesthetics.

While neither of these visions "solves" the numerous problems and issues surrounding motherhood, both texts are important in exploring the psychological issue of maternal subjectivity through the social issues of class and race. For example, black feminists such as Patricia Hill Collins have criticized white feminism for minimizing the importance of race and class in theorizing motherhood. The case of Peterkin is useful in illuminating the complexity of racial issues to maternal subjectivity, especially for southern women, where race has always been fore-grounded. Most discussions of race and motherhood look at the mother's own race; Peterkin illuminates, however, that the combination of con-structions of white femininity with white *perceptions* of the femininity of racial Others can also be crucial to (white) maternal subjectivity. Where Newman underscores the binary of male=mind, female=body, Peterkin, in keeping with the traditional white southern dichotomy of "pure" white ladies versus sensuous and "loose" black women, displaces the mind-body dichotomy from male-female to white-black. Her exam-ple illustrates how including race in theorizing maternal subjectivity hopelessly tangles any easy binary oppositions. *The Hard-Boiled Virgin,* on the other hand, provides glimmers of insight into the complex rela-tionship between class position and maternal identity. Newman's text suggests that class differences in maternal subjectivity can stem not only from material considerations but from less concrete differences as well, such as a woman's attitudes towards her own class privilege. Finally, the fact that both texts are deeply southern in their outlook also indicates that future researchers in the area of maternal subjectivity might profit from further study of regional differences among American women.

Notes

1. See the review essays on maternity and motherhood by Ellen Ross and Alice Adams for excellent summaries of the recent trends in feminist scholar-ship.

2. Judith Leavitt documents the overwhelming commonalities of women's experiences of labor throughout American history. Over and over, they "recounted their trials with wrenching repetitiveness" (159), repeating themes

of being "so miserable," "at death's door," "at the point of death," and so forth (159). Indeed, many were at death's door, since "death remained a persistent threat and a too-common reality in the years before the 1930s and 1940s, when America's maternal mortality rates finally began to fall" (Leavitt 159). And rather than being in less danger than white women, women of color actually died far more frequently than did whites. "Between 1900 and 1935 approximately sixty white women and over a hundred nonwhite women died for every ten thousand live births" (Leavitt 160).

3. She may be referring to the Sheppard-Towner Maternity and Infancy Act of 1921. It subsidized midwife education programs, mainly in the Southern States.

6

MATERNAL CONCEPTIONS
IN TONI MORRISON'S *THE BLUEST EYE* AND *TAR BABY:*
"A WOMAN HAS TO BE A DAUGHTER
BEFORE SHE CAN BE ANY KIND OF WOMAN"

Andrea O'Reilly

"There was something so valuable about what happened when one became a mother. For me it was the most liberating thing that ever happened. . . ."[1] In this statement Morrison defines mothering, in the words of Donna Bassin, Margaret Honey, and Meryle Mahrer Kaplan, "as a freeing, generative experience" (2). Such a view, they emphasize, contrasts sharply with "the predominant image of the mother in white Western society [which assumes mothers are] ever-bountiful, ever-giving, self-sacrificing . . . not destroyed or overwhelmed by the demands of [their] child[ren]" (2-3).[2] Motherhood is a central theme in Morrison's fiction and is a topic she returns to time and time again in her many interviews and articles. In her reflections on motherhood, both inside and outside her fiction, Morrison articulates a fully developed theory of African American mothering which is central to her larger political and philosophical stance on black womanhood in America. The aim of this chapter is to delineate Morrison's theory of mothering, and to detail how initiation into motherhood and perspectives on maternity in *The Bluest Eye* and *Tar Baby* enact and represent Morrison's maternal philosophy.

Black women, Toni Morrison commented in an *Essence* interview

[need to] pay attention to the ancient proprieties—which for me means the ability to be "the ship" and the "safe harbour." Our history as Black women is the history of women who could build a house and have some children *and* there was no problem. What we have known is how to be complete human beings, so that we did not let education keep us from our nurturing abilities . . . To lose that is to diminish ourselves unnecessarily. It is not a question, it's not a conflict. You don't have to give up anything. You *choose* your responsibilities. (135)[3]

In a conversation with Gloria Naylor, Morrison elaborates further:

[T]he point is that freedom is choosing your responsibility; it's choosing the ones you want . . . A lady doctor has to be able to say, "I want to go home." And the one at home has the right to say, "I want to go to medical school." That's all there is to that, but then the choices cause problems where there are no problems because "either/or" seems to set up the conflict, first in the language and then in life. . . . I tried hard to be both the ship and the safe harbor at the same time, to be able to make a house and be on the job market and still nurture the children. . . . No one should be asked to make a choice between a home or a career. Why not have both? It's all possible. (195, 197)[4]

In these two statements Morrison constructs a very specific definition of black womanhood.[5] Black women, according to Morrison, are providers and nurturers; they inhabit the public sphere of work and the private realm of home and do so unproblematically; they are both "ship and safe harbour, inn and trail." Her emphasis upon responsibility makes commitment to kin and community central to her definition of black womanhood as well. Morrison's view of black womanhood is most fully developed in the black mammy figure. She explains:

[I]f women are to become full, complete the answer may not be in the future, but the answer may be back there. And that does interest me more than the fully liberated woman, the woman who understands her past, not the woman who merely has her way. Because that woman did know how to nurture, *and* survive. . . . [I]t seems to me that the most respectable person is that woman who is a healer and understands plants and stones and yet they live in the world. Those people are always strange, when they get to the city. These women know what time it is by looking at the sky. I don't want to reduce it to some sort of heavy know-how, but it's paying attention to different sets of information, and that information certainly isn't useful in terms of a career . . . It's a quality that normally one associates with a mammy, a black mammy. She could nurse, she could heal, she could chop wood, she could do all those things. And that's always been a pejorative word, a bad thing, but it isn't. That stereotype is bad only when people think it's less . . . Those women were terrific, but they were perceived of as beastly in the very things that were wonderful about them. (81-82)[6]

With the black mammy figure we see the full embodiment of the "ancient properties" of black womanhood: as "chopper of wood" and "healer of the sick" she achieves a symmetry of love and work; in her commitment to history over the self—the woman who understands her past, not merely the woman who has her way—she embraces the communal responsibility so valued by Morrison.

In her article "The Convergence of Feminism and Ethnicity in the Fiction of Toni Morrison," Denard argues that "[black women] always maintained whether they desire it or not a connection to their ethnic community. They are the 'cultural bearers,' they function as a parent . . . as a sort of umbrella figure in the community not just with [their] children but with all children" (174). The expression "ancient properties," in Morrison, is thus a shorthand signifier for a woman who defines herself in connection with her African American culture and history, and who serves as an ambassador for her people, bringing the past to the present and keeping African American culture in the community of black people. To have the ancient properties is to live life according to the ways of the foremothers; it is to define oneself according to the script of traditional black womanhood.

Morrison, thus, does not endorse the existentialist or power feminism championed by much of Anglo-American feminism. The feminist stance that Morrison advocates is an ethnic and cultural one. Carolyn Denard explains:

Among black women, who have historically suffered oppression because of both race and gender, there is usually a simultaneous concern for both these issues. They abhor both sexist and racist oppression. But because of their minority ethnic status, which keeps their allegiance to ancestral group foremost, they shun an advocacy of the kind of political, existential feminism embraced by many women of the majority culture. For black women, their concern with feminism is usually more group-centred than self-centred, more cultural than political. As a result, they tend to be concerned more with the particular female cultural values of their own ethnic group rather than with those of women in general. They advocate what may be termed ethnic cultural feminism. (171-72)

In Morrison's fiction women who shun the ancient properties of ethnic cultural feminism and embrace Anglo-American definitions of feminism, do not achieve, what Morrison calls, "complete[ness]" and "full[ness]" of self. These qualities are obtained only by those women who live their lives according to the ancient properties of their foremothers.

Morrison's fiction details a particular way of being modelled on the ancient ways and values of the foremothers and positions the motherline as the way by which the ancient path is followed and passed on generationally. Connecting to the motherline, the young woman learns and claims for herself the ancient properties of her foremothers. Morrison argues further that the ancient properties are at the core of black women's empowerment. Women, Naomi Lowinsky writes in *Stories from the Motherline,* are cut off from their motherline, and "[have] paid a terrible price for cutting [them]selves off from [their] feminine roots" (26). What is lost, she emphasizes, is female authenticity and authority. Morrison advances a similar argument: fullness and completeness of being are assured only by living in accordance with the ancient properties. In Morrison's writing, daughters need mothers to become women and mothers need women to stay daughters. In an interview with Bessie W. Jones and Audrey Vinson, Morrison argues that: "A woman has to be a daughter before she can be any kind of woman. If she doesn't know how to relate to her ancestors, to her tribe, so to speak, she is not good for much" (184).[7]

One could argue that the main theme of Morrison's fiction is summed up in her oft-cited quotation: "When you kill the ancestor you kill yourself. I want to point out the dangers, to show that nice things don't always happen to the totally self reliant if there is no historical connection"[8] "From the outset of her literary career," critic Angelita Reyes emphasizes, "Toni Morrison has been deeply concerned with the preservation of black folklore, and with sustaining positive black cultural values" (19). Speaking specifically of Morrison's fourth novel *Tar Baby*, but applicable to all of her writings, Reyes maintains that what Morrison asks is that "black people . . . not lose sight of their [African American] consciousness" (19). In a conversation with Elsie B. Washington, Toni Morrison comments:

[Grandparents and ancestors are] DNA, it's where you get your information, your cultural information. Also it's your protection, it's your education. They were responsible *for* us, and we have to be responsible *to* them. . . . You can't just *take*. And if you ignore that, you put yourself in a spiritually dangerous position of being self-sufficient, having no group that you're dependent on. (238)[9]

Historical connection and communal identification, for Morrison, are absolutely essential for the psychological well-being of African Americans. The women of the ancient properties are the ones who both embody and carry that ancestral memory, they are the cultural bearers and the cultural translators. In Morrison's fiction, Barbara Hill Rigney writes, "women are the primary tale-tellers and the transmitters of history, as well as the singing teachers" (10). Trudier Harris describes these women as "keepers of the tradition" and "culture bearers . . . they are women who have kept their funkiness intact" (41). "These women are free," Harris continues, "but the freedom they experience is one wrought in nurturing their children and grandchildren, not in defiance and destruction of them" (40). Speaking to Nellie McKay about her ancestors, Morrison commented: "What is uppermost in my mind . . . is that my life seems to be dominated by information about black women. They were the culture bearers, and they told us [children] what to do . . ." (140).[10] "Black women," critic Karla Holloway writes, "carry the voice of the mother—they are the progenitors, the assurance of the line" (123). "[Women] as carriers of the voice," Holloway continues, "carry wisdom —mother wit. They teach the children to survive and remember" (123).

The Bluest Eye is concerned with a mother's loss of the ancient properties and the devastating consequences of such for herself and her daughter. Of interest to Morrison in this, her first novel, are how women become disinherited from their motherline through assimilation in the dominant culture and the impact of this on women's ability to mother. Pauline Breedlove's disconnection from her motherline renders her incapable of nurturing and sustaining her daughter, Pecola. Pauline's failed mothering, though apparent throughout the text, is signified most powerfully by Pauline's inability to love her daughter upon her birth. This "failure to bond," to paraphrase the medical diagnosis, becomes in *The Bluest Eye* the central trope of the loss of maternal nurturance engendered by assimilation and the resulting displacement of the motherline.

Much critical commentary on the novel has centred on the primer which opens the text and introduces each chapter. The primer presents the ideal family: in "the very pretty house" live Dick and Jane with their "nice" mother and "big and strong" father.[11] This white middle-class nuclear family of the primer is scripted as the normal and real family arrangement. Families are measured by this ideal and are encouraged to emulate it. The "Dick and Jane" family, however, is available only to a select few. Families like the Breedloves in *The Bluest Eye* can never be a Dick and Jane family though such families will continually aspire to achieve the ideal and forever measure their own selves against it.

The primer's construction of the ideal family enacts the complex relationship between subjectivity, discourse, and ideology. The function of the primer in the educational system is to teach young students how to read. However, in acquiring literacy the student learns more than language; he or she internalizes the values of the text that is read. In the instance of the primer while the student learns the workings of nouns and verbs, he or she is also inscribed in the dominant ideology of the family. Critic Donald Gibson elaborates:

[T]he act of learning to read and write means exposure to the values of the culture for which the reading material emanates. If one wants to read or write, then one must pay for the privilege. The cost of learning to read and write carried with it the necessity to submit to values beyond and other than literacy per se, for words do not exist independent of value. One cannot learn to read without being subjected to the values engraved in the text.[12]

Gibson's concept here of the "enact[ment] [of] self-oppression" through the internalization of the dominant culture's values echoes Louis Althusser's theory of hailing and interpellation. Kaja Silverman explains in her *Subject of Semiotics:*

Althusser helps us to understand that discourse may also consist of an exchange between a person and a cultural agent . . . (Althusser isolates priests and education as particularly important cultural agents). The agent addresses the person, and in the process defines not so much its own as the other's identity . . . Althusser refers to the address as "hailing," and its successful outcome as "interpellation." "Interpellation" occurs when the person to whom the agent speaks recognizes him or herself in that speech, and takes up subjective residence there. (48-49)

However, the subject position the primer offers lies in sharp contrast to the lived realities of the Breedlove family. Yet, following Althusser, the text's subject becomes not only more preferable but also more real; it is internalized. One's real, own lived life becomes, in the words of Pauline, "like the after thoughts one has just before sleep, the early-morning and late evenings edges of her day, the dark edges that made the daily life with the Fishers lighter, more delicate, more lovely" (101). The real, however, does frequently interrupt and disrupt the assumed subjectivity; as with Pauline's tooth, the lived/actual often shatters the illusion.[13]

In a 1978 film interview Morrison commented; "I suppose *The Bluest Eye* is about one's dependency on the world for identification, self value, feelings or worth."[14] In *The Bluest Eye* the original self is displaced through interpellation. As Karen Carmean observes, "[Pauline] conform[s] to a role defined by others, and in confusing self with role, Pauline denies any possibility of growth. [She] represents many, who, in adopting white values and standards of behaviour, deny their own essential value, substituting false—even destructive—standards" (21). Critics of *The Bluest Eye,* however, have not considered why Pauline, and later Pecola, are so easily seduced by that master narrative of beauty and romance, while other characters, like the McTeers, remain relatively indifferent to it. Pauline's life lacked the essence necessary to, in the words of the text, "stand erect and spit the misery out on the street instead [of holding] it in where it could lap into her" because in her identification with the dominant white culture she is severed from her motherline (61).

In her brilliant piece, "Eruptions of Funk: Historicizing Toni Morrison," Susan Willis contends that: "the problem at the center of Morrison's writing is how to maintain an Afro-American cultural heritage once the relationship to the black rural south has been stretched thin over distance and generations" (264). As a young girl in Alabama, Pauline's life was, literally, full of colour: "My whole dress was messed with purple, and it never did wash out. Not the dress nor me. I could feel that purple deep inside me. And that lemonade Mama used to make when Papa came out of the fields. It be cool and yellowish. . . . And that streak of green them June bugs made on the trees" (92). Down home "all of them colors was in [her]" (92). Newly married, she and Cholly move north to Ohio where Pauline experienced, in the words of the text "the lonesomest time of [her] life" (93). Pauline talks about how with moving north "everything changed": "It was hard to get to know folks up here, and I missed my people. I weren't used to so much white folks" (93). The few women she meets snicker at her way of talking and are amused by her unstraightened hair (94). Alone and lonely Pauline turns to her husband Cholly, in the words of the text, for "reassurance, entertainment, for things to fill the vacant places" (93). It would seem that cultural dislocation, and the resulting alienation from one's heritage and family, are at the heart of Pauline's emotional estrangement which drives her to the movies and eventually leads her to a hatred of her black self. Alienated from her rural culture and assimilated in the values of the dominant one, Pauline loses what is called in *The Bluest Eye* "funkiness": "the . . . funkiness of passion, the funkiness of nature, the funkiness of the wide range of emotions" (68). In Morrison's writing, funkiness signifies the black cultural identity which is lost through assimilation to white bourgeois culture. Disconnected from her motherline, Pauline has lost her funkiness and the ancient properties that would have grounded her in the values of her people and enabled her to resist interpellation and fashion an authentic selfhood. "Having no people" Pauline is rendered vulnerable to the seductive myths of the dominant white culture (147).

Pauline's relationship with her daughter Pecola, her second child, is initially described as caring and close mother-child attachment. "That second time [pregnant]" Pauline says, "I felt good and wasn't thinking on the carrying, just on the baby itself. I used to talk to it whilst it be still in the womb. Like good friends we was" (98). "Up til the end," Pauline tells us, "(she) felt good about that baby" (99). She also says that "[she'd] love it no matter what it looked like" (98). Once born, the daughter is described as a "big old healthy thing" (99) and is perceived by her mother as a bright and quick child: "They gave her to me for a nursing, and she liked to pull my nipple off right away. She caught on fast . . . A right smart baby she was" (99-100). Pauline is also attracted to, and fascinated by, her newly born daughter: "I used to like to watch her. . . . Eyes all soft and wet. A cross between a puppy and a dying man" (100). Although, Pauline is impressed by her daughter's health and quickness, and is mesmerized by her facial features, she sees her daughter as ugly: "I knowed she was ugly. Head full of pretty hair, but Lord she was ugly" (100). Pauline cannot find in her real flesh-and-blood daughter the unborn child of her imagination: "She looked so different from what I thought. Reckin I talked to it so much I conjured up a mind's eye view of it" (99). Since Pauline spent much of her pregnancy in movie houses, the text suggests her "mind's eye view" of the unborn child was formed in terms of white definitions of beauty and acceptability. The child imagined in the womb is light skinned, fine featured, but the real Pecola is born very dark.

Pauline's birth experience also contributes to Pauline's perception of her daughter as ugly. For the birth of her second child Pauline chooses a hospital over a home birth "so [she] could be easeful" (98). Ironically, though not surprisingly, Pauline's hospital birth is anything but easeful. As a poor, black woman Pauline is treated with contempt and indifference by the medical staff; in the hospital the doctors talk "nice friendly talk" to the white women, but they do not speak to Pauline nor make eye contact with her. To the doctors she is merely "[one] of these here women . . . [who] deliver right away and with no pain. Just like horses" (99), "the primitive woman" who, as Tess Cosslett explains in *Women Writing Childbirth,* is said to give birth without discomfort or inconvenience. While Pauline resists this racist categorization and the denial of her subjectivity and the dehumanization of her birth experience on which it is predicated by forcing one doctor to look her in the eye and by "moan[ing] something awful . . . to let them know having a baby was more than a bowel movement" (99), her self perception is, nonetheless, structured through the degradation of her labour experience. So when her child is born, and it is both black and female, Pauline sees it as she herself was seen while in labour as undesirable, irrelevant and unimportant. Significantly, when Pauline attempts to convey her surprise at seeing her actual daughter, in contrast to the image of her while pregnant, she does so by way of analogy to her own mother and herself as daughter: "So when I seed it, it was like looking at a picture of your mama when she was a girl. You knows who she is, but she don't look the same" (99). This analogy invokes the theme of the need for the parents to love themselves if they are to love their children. At the movies and while in labour, Pauline learns that her blackness renders her undesirable; it therefore is not surprising that when Pauline holds her very black daughter in her arms she perceives her as ugly.

The Bluest Eye exemplifies the need for mothers to maintain a strong authentic self so that they may nurture the same in their daughters. In her article appropriately entitled, "Difficult Survival: Mothers and Daughters in *The Bluest Eye*," Joyce Pettis argues that Pauline fails at nurturing her daughter because she herself is unnurtured. Quoting Adrienne Rich from *Of Woman Born,* Pettis writes; "The nurture of daughters in a patriarchy calls for a strong sense of self-nurture in the mother" (27). Disconnected from her motherline, Pauline is rendered vulnerable to interpellation in the dominant white supremacist ideology which results in the effacement and disparagement of her black female self. "It is not simply," to quote Rich again, "that . . . mothers feel both responsible and powerless. It is that they carry their own guilt and self-hatred over into their daughters' experiences" (244). This generational continuation of female self-hatred explains and is signified by Pauline's inability to love her black female child upon her birth. Cynthia Davis has written that in *The Bluest Eye,* as in Morrison's later writings, there "is [no] sense of history available to women, and without it they have neither the models nor the contextual information to make themselves whole" (22). They have no motherline or foremothers with whom to identify. While this point is arguable with respect to Morrison's later writings, it seems accurate for *The Bluest Eye*. Having abandoned her maternal culture, Pauline is disconnected from her motherline and thus lacks the ancient properties that would afford her a strong sense of self and enable her to embrace her daughter upon her birth.

As with *The Bluest Eye* Morrison's fourth's novel *Tar Baby* details a woman's disconnection from her motherline; however, in this instance the woman, Jadine, is a daughter whose disconnection from the motherline results not in a failure of mothering as with Pauline, but in an inability to achieve the authentic selfhood of black womanhood championed by Morrison. In *The Bluest Eye* Pauline becomes disconnected from her motherline in and through her internalization of the values of the dominant culture and this explains and is signified by her inability to mother her daughter upon her birth. Jadine's disconnection from the motherline is occasioned by the death of her mother and results in her disavowal of the ancient proprieties of black womanhood that would afford her an authentic selfhood. As with *The Bluest Eye* this narrative of disconnection and loss is enacted and signified through the female reproductive experience; Pauline's inability to love Pecola enacts her estrangement from the motherline, Jadine's dread and loathing of motherhood, particularly as it is represented by the fecund maternal body, depicts her disconnection and is what gives rise to her sense of inauthenticity and incompleteness

The central theme of *Tar Baby,* critic Angelita Reyes argues, may be summed up in Therese's warning to Son: "[D]on't go to L'Arbe de la Croix. . . forget her [Jadine]. There is nothing in her Parts for you. She has forgotten her ancient properties" (305). This novel asks, in Reyes's words, that "Black people . . . not lose sight of their African consciousness" (19). Thus, Tar Baby can be interpreted, as critic Marilyn Sanders Mobley observes, "as a modern cautionary tale in which Morrison draws on the Afro-American oral narrative tradition to expose the pitfalls of white middle-class aspirations for the black woman and to illustrate the consequences of her social and cultural misbehaviour" (285). The moral story or fable that Tar Baby tells is specifically gendered: a woman, Jadine, rejects the ancient properties of traditional black womanhood and adopts the values of the dominant white culture. This rejection causes psychic fragmentation, or in Mobley's words, a "divided consciousness" (285). *Tar Baby* tells the story of Jadine's quest for wholeness and its ultimate failure. Mobley attributes Jadine's failure to her "reject[ionl [of] the very cultural constructions of race and mothering that could heal her and transform her consciousness" (285-86).

The novel opens with Morrison's dedication to her foremothers: "For [my foremothers] . . . and each of their sisters—and each of their sisters, all of whom knew their true and ancient properties." The phrase "ancient properties" frames the novel: it occurs in the dedication and it is mentioned by Therese on the penultimate page of the novel. We enter the text through this dedication and it acts as our moral point of reference for our interpretation and judgement of the novel. "The women of the dedication—grandmother, mother, aunts, and sister of [Morrison]," Eleanor W. Traylor writes, "are . . . the guides to whom the narrative of the writer is accountable" (149). We realize upon coming to know Jadine that she has, in Karla Holloway's words, "den[ied] [her] lineage. Instead of Jadine having an inherent self as a Black woman, she has chosen to dispossess herself" (120). Significantly, we first encounter Jadine as a disembodied voice overheard by an unidentified man. Her entry into the narrative suggests her alienation and isolation. Her voice and words reinforce this sense of herself: "warm on the inside, cold at the edges, or was it the other way around?" "I'm never lonely. Never" (6). In contrast to the dedication, this disembodied voice does not speak the ancient properties of community and ancestry. Hers is not the voice of the foremothers honoured on the opening page of the text. In an interview in *Essence* magazine, Morrison says of Jadine:

She has lost the tar quality, the ability to hold something together that otherwise would fall apart—which is what I mean by the nurturing ability. That's what one surrenders or can surrender in order to do this other thing—in order to go and get a degree in art history, learn four languages and be in the movies and stuff. That sounds like I'm putting it down: I'm not. I'm saying that the point is to be able to do both. (131)[16]

In contrast, the woman in yellow whom Jadine sees in the market comes to signify and embody those ancient properties:

The vision itself was a woman much too tall. Under her canary yellow dress was too much hip, too much bust. The agency would laugh her out of the lobby, so why was she and everybody else in the store transfixed? The height? The skin like tar against the canary yellow dress? . . . . Two upside down-V's were scored into each of her cheeks, her hair was wrapped in a gelee as yellow as her dress. . . . The woman leaned into the dairy section and opened a carton from which she selected three eggs. Then she put her right elbow into the palm of her left hand and held the eggs aloft between earlobe and shoulder. She looked up then and they saw something in her eyes so powerful it had burnt away the eyelashes. (45)

This image of the African woman in the yellow dress is used by Morrison, critic Barbara Christian argues, "as a symbol for the authenticity that the jaded Jadine lacks" (244). The defiant stance of the woman's body, as Christian observes, is a manifestation of "the woman's inner strength, beauty, and pride" (144). The woman's Africaness is inscribed in the Vs on her cheeks, while her fertility, like that of Pilate in Morrison's earlier novel *Song of Solomon,* is signified by the eggs she carries in the curve of her neck. Her beauty, as Jadine tells us, is "unphotographical"(46). She, unlike the Cover girl model Jadine, cannot be represented or appropriated by the discourse of white culture. The power which Jadine tells us burnt her lashes is the power of the ancient properties of black womanhood. The woman in yellow, Morrison explained in a conversation with Gloria Naylor, "is somehow transcendent and whatever she really was, what she was perceived as by Jadine, is the real chic. The one that authenticates everything. The one that is very clear in some deep way about her womanhood."[17] She represents, Morrison explains further, "a complete individual who owns herself. . . . She is the original self."[18]

In Morrison's fiction the colour yellow, in particular yellow dresses, signify the original black female self of the ancient properties. Creole-speaking Rochelle in Toni Morrison's second novel, *Sula,* wears a canary yellow dress and, like the woman in yellow who had "burnt away eye lashes," Rochelle "rubbed burned matches over her eyes" (28). Son, the character whom many critics interpret as Jadine's foil because he embraces, while she denies, the ancient properties, dreams of "yellow houses with white doors which women opened and shouted 'Come on in, you honey!'" (6). He attempts to make his dream become Jadine's: "[While Jadine slept, Son] inserts his dream of yellow houses into hers" (119).

Jadine, like the other shoppers in the market, is mesmerized by the "transcendent beauty" (46) of the African woman: "She would deny it now, but along with everybody else in the market, Jadine gasped. Just a little. Just a sudden intake of air. Just a quick snatch of breath before that woman's woman—that mother/sister/she: that unphotographable beauty —took it all away" (46). The African woman, as Samuels and Hudson-Weems observe, "make[s] Jade confront her cultural heritage" (80). However, when this African woman finally does make eye contact with the spellbound Jadine, she "looked right at Jadine . . . and, with a small parting of her lips, shot an arrow of saliva between her teeth down to the pavement and the hearts below" (46). The African woman is disgusted by Jadine for she sees in her a black woman who has repudiated her ancient proprieties.

"The woman's insulting gesture," the narrator tells us, "derailed [Jadine]—shaken her out of proportion to the incident. Why had she wanted that woman to like and respect her? It had certainly taken the zing out of the magazine cover as well as her degree" (47). "The woman," Jadine later reflects, "made her feel lonely in a way. Lonely and inauthentic" (48). Jadine's realization signals the beginning of her spiritual quest. "[T]he vision [which] materialized in a yellow dress" functions as an epiphany which awakens Jadine to her inauthenticity (46). Jadine's position is at the threshold of the second stage of the spiritual quest, the moment of awakening. Jadine has been awakened to the nothingness of her life and is able now to reconnect back to her motherline and reclaim her ancient properties. Significantly, the crisis of self-definition caused by the sight of the yellow woman is configured in racial terms. Jadine questions whether she should marry her white lover and wonders "if the person he wants to marry is me or a black girl?" (48). "And then," the narrator tells us, "she ran away because Ryk is white and the woman spit at her and she had to come to see her aunt and uncle . . ." (48).

Shortly after Jadine returns to Isle des Chevaliers she meets Son Green. The text presents, and most readers interpret, Son as the embodiment of essential African American funkiness. Later, it is the mythic tree women, the fecund women of the motherline, who attempt to rescue Jadine and return her to her ancient properties:

They were delighted when first they saw her, thinking a runaway child had been restored to them. But looking closer they saw differently. This girl was fighting to get away from them. The women hanging from the trees were quiet now, but arrogant—mindful as they were of their values, their exceptional femaleness: knowing as they did that the first world of the world had been built with their sacred properties: that they alone could hold together the stones of pyramids and the rushes of Moses's crib: knowing their steady consistency, their pace of glaciers, their permanent embrace, they wondered at the girl's desperate struggle down below to be free, to be something other then they were. (183)

Jadine, Karla Holloway argues, "is called by the goddess earth who embodies the cosmic life principle. Rejecting the call of the trees, she is cut off from the good consciousness—knowledge of the mother" (118). "Jadine's womanhood," Holloway continues, "is seriously in question in the face of these ancient females who have not lost touch with who they are . . . and understand their primal connection to this archetype" (119). Jadine resists the pull of the tar by dancing with the tree in what is portrayed as a heterosexual embrace: "Press together like man and wife" (183). Jadine is finally able to pull herself from the swamp when "her right knee grazed something hard and she managed to lift her leg and bend it enough to kneel on the hard thing that seemed to be growing out of her partner the tree" (183). The phallic imagery of this passage does, to pardon the pun, noticeably stick out: the "hard thing growing out of the tree" suggests a male erection. Thus it would seem, as Holloway suggests, "that [Jadine] kneels on masculinity and uses it to pull herself out of the earth's tar baby's clutch rather than to identify and to complete her being. This pull toward individuation . . . [separating from the tar women] becomes the basis of her loss" (119). More specifically, Jadine identifies with male sexuality rather than female fertility as represented by the tree women and the tar. In a 1981 interview with Thomas LeClair, Morrison elaborated upon the symbolic significance of tar in African mythology:

Tar seemed to me to be an odd thing to be in Western story, and I found that there is a tar lady in African mythology . . . At one time, a tar pit was a holy place, at least an important place, because tar was used to build things. It came naturally out of the earth: it held together things like Moses's little boat and the pyramids. For me, the tar baby came to mean the black woman who can hold things together. (122)

Morrison's discussion makes sense out of the tree women's statement that they helped build Moses' crib and the pyramids. These women are the tar ladies of African mythology who used the sacred properties of the tar to build civilizations. They are the women of the ancient properties who both build and create, who are ship and harbour. Jadine's problem is that she cannot imagine doing both; for her being a ship and harbour are mutually exclusive. "[He] wanted her to settle for wifely competence when she could be almighty, to settle for fertility rather than originality, nurturing instead of building" (269).

In Eloe at Rosie's, Jadine sleeps in a "little bedroom without windows" (123). Windowless and with two doors, one to the living room and one that opened to the back yard, this room suggests a womb-like environment. Significantly, Jadine finds the room "suffocating" (123). To get some air Jadine goes outside only to confront "the blackest nothing she had ever seen. . . . It's not possible she thought, for anything to be this black" (251). Jadine's unease with the closeness of the room and the darkness outside symbolically marks her rejection of motherhood and the ancient properties of black womanhood. Significantly, Jadine inscribes blackness as feminine: "She might as well have been in a cave, a grave, the dark womb of the earth, suffocating with the sound of plant life moving, but deprived of its sight" (252). In *Tar Baby* as in *Song of Solomon,* the ancient properties of black womanhood are positioned in opposition to both maleness and whiteness. Jadine fears the former and aspires to be the latter. Pointedly, the text concludes with Jadine returning to Paris—emblematic of white/masculinist discourse—feeling "lean and male" (275).

Jadine's rejection of the ancient properties, specifically her fear of the maternal is represented in this text by the night women who visit Jadine in the black womb. When she asks: "What do you want with me . . . ?" they reply: "They looked as though they had just been waiting for that question and they each pulled out a breast and showed it to her. . . . They just stood around in the room, jostling each other gently . . . revealing one breast and then two . . . (258). To this Jadine responds: "'I have breasts too,' she said or thought or willed, 'I have breasts too'" (258). However, the night women do not, in the words of the text, "believe her. They just held their own higher and pushed their own farther out and looked at her. All of them revealing both their breasts except the woman in yellow. She did something more shocking—she stretched out a long arm and showed Jadine her three big eggs" (258-59). Jadine's rejection of the maternal is clear. The reasons for it, however, are not—leaving much space for critical speculation and debate. Critic Peter Erickson attributes Jadine's fear to her inability to see motherhood as compatible with a career. He writes: "The novel does not allow [Jadine's] avoidance of motherhood to be perceived sympathetically, yet the maternal issue presents itself in the form of a conflict between mutually exclusive imperatives" (305). "In the novel," Erickson continues, "there is little suggestion that Jadine could, with complete dignity, choose only 'originality' and 'building.' There is also little suggestion that she could have both 'nurturing' and 'building'" (305). Women in Morrison do both build and nurture, but Jadine herself did not know such women because she grew up on the "Streets" separated from her black community.

Jadine attempts, as Karla Holloway argues, "to exist without a discovery of 'whose' child she is" (119). "She has chosen to dispossess herself" (120). Although an orphan, Holloway emphasizes, "Jadine had warmth and protection offered her through her extended family, her aunt and uncle" (190). Ondine and Sydney are, according to Holloway, "black folk" who maintain a strong sense of racial identity despite their isolation on Isle de Chevaliers (123). Ondine, in particular, attempts to impart to Jadine her ancient properties. "Women like Ondine," Holloway contends, "are mothers and daughters and are connected in this way to things past and future" (123). I would argue, however, that Ondine does not, as the expression goes, practice what she preaches. Although she espouses black folk values, she identifies with the bourgeois white lifestyle of the Streets. As Samuels and Hudson-Weems observe: "Unlike Pilate, who passes the legacy of her cultural heritage to her nephew Milkman, Ondine does not perform this function for Jadine" (83). She does not provide the example of folk caring and loving that she talks about. "Ondine," Samuels and Hudson-Weems continue, "seems far more interested in the welfare and care of white culture than in [her] own [life]" (83). As Ondine says: "I know my Kitchens. Better than I know my face" (39). And Ondine and Sydney, though well meaning, orphan Jadine a second time when they give her over to the "Streets."

However, Ondine is right when she says to Jadine: "A girl has got to be a daughter first. She have to learn that. And if she never learns how to be a daughter, she can't never learn how to be a woman . . . [A] real woman: a woman good enough for a child: good enough for a man—good enough even for the respect of other women" (281). What Ondine does not realize until Jadine is grown is that she has not been that mother to Jadine; she has not replaced the mother Jadine lost. Ondine says to Jadine: "I never told you nothing. I never told you nothing at all and I take full responsibility for that. But I have to tell you something now" (281). Ondine, I think, has come to realize that in wanting more for her niece she has alienated Jadine from the black community, and more specifically, has severed Jadine's connection to the motherline.

When Ondine later tells Jadine: "You didn't have a mother long enough" (281), she identifies the source of Jadine's general malaise and her specific anxiety about motherhood. In Morrison mothering is essential for the psychological well-being of children because it connects the child to the motherline and imparts the ancient properties. Hudson-Weems and Samuels contend that "Jadine's status as an orphan is significant . . . [at] the crucial age of twelve, a point of transition from childhood to adolescence, she is deprived of parents to nurture and guide her" (83). Jadine loses her mother at precisely the time when a girl becomes a woman.

In Baltimore before her mother's death Jadine comes upon a dog in heat on the streets. She tells us that:

the retired postman [came out] and crack[ed] the bitch over the back and sen[t] her home, she who had done nothing but be "in heat" which she couldn't help but which was her fault just the same so it was she who was beaten and cracked over the head and spine with the mop handle and made to run away and I felt sorry for her and went looking for her to see if she was hurt and when I found her . . . another dog sniffed her ass embarrassing me in the sunlight. (124)

From this, Jadine resolves to "never let the hunger show" (125). "She decided then and there at the age of twelve in Baltimore never to be broken in the hands of any man" (124). "And anybody who wanted nice from this colored girl would have to get it with pliers and chloroform, because Never" (124). Significantly, immediately after this scene, we are told of the mother's death. "When her mother died and she went to Philadelphia and then away to school, she was so quick to learn . . . but not smile, because Never . . . [B]eneath the easy manners was a claw ready to rein in the dogs, because Never" (124). Jadine represses the sexual in her self because for her it represents shame and a loss of control. Jadine's repression of the sexual and sensual thus signifies her denial of the ancient properties. The structural juxtaposition of the story about the dogs and the mention of the mother's death suggest that her denial of sexuality, specifically, and the ancient properties in general, is linked to her mother's death.

The bitch in heat is struck and the mother dies in Jadine's twelfth year, at the threshold of womanhood. Jadine's fear and denial of her developing sexuality may have been negotiated had her mother lived. But without a mother, Jadine is left to enter womanhood alone and unguided. Jade at the age of twelve, is twice orphaned, first by her mother's death and then by being sent off to school and handed over to the Streets. This severs Jade from her motherline and occasions her rejection of the ancient properties and repudiation of the maternal. Jadine's fears about sexuality and intimacy and her rejection of motherhood stems from the loss of her mother and her disconnection from the motherline. Sexuality and motherhood are problematic for Jadine. She had no one there to teach her how to be a woman and become a mother. Orphaned at twelve, and failed by Ondine who mothered her in ways of assimilation rather than resistance, Jadine must find her own way. Ondine tells Jadine: "You don't need your own natural mother to be a daughter" (281). But you do, I would suggest, need a mother who protects and fosters a daughter's female and black self by keeping the daughter connected to the motherline. Ondine does not instill in Jadine the ancient properties that would have empowered her as she grew into womanhood. As she says to Jadine: "I thought I was doing right by sending you to all them schools and so I never told you and I should have" (281). Ondine's realization, however, comes too late (264).

The Bluest Eye and *Tar Baby* enact and affirm Morrison's theory of the empowerment of women through the motherline by detailing the tragedies of *dis*connection: Pauline cannot love her self or her daughter; Jadine shuns that which would give meaning to her life. This story of disconnection and loss is narrated though the inability to mother, Pauline, and the avoidance of motherhood, Jadine. This denial of maternity is signified in Pauline's rejection of her newly born daughter and, with Jadine, in the disdain with which she holds motherhood generally and the fecund maternal body in particular. In and through Jadine and Pauline's repudiation of motherhood and their motherline, Morrison affirms their centrality to black women's politics of empowerment; in her words, " a woman has to be a daughter before she can be any kind of woman."

Notes

1. Toni Morrison, Interview with Bill Moyers, *Conversations with Toni Morrison,* ed. Danille Taylor-Guthrie (Jackson: U of Mississippi P, 1994) 270-71.

2. Their critique is typical of feminist thought in the 1970s. As one mother described motherhood: "I know that when my children are small they need me. But sometimes I think I'll go nuts if I don't get out of this house and meet some grown ups. I find I'm starting to talk like a three-year old all the time now," from Meg Luxton's *More Than a Labour of Love* (Toronto: Women's Press, 1980) 87.

3. Interview with Judith Wilson, (1981), *Conversations with Toni Morrison* 129-37.

4. (1985), *Conversations with Toni Morrison* 188-217. In her early article, "What the Black Woman Thinks About Women's Lib," Morrison argued that "[the] black woman had nothing to fall back on: not maleness, not whiteness, not ladyhood, not anything. And out of that profound desolation of her reality she may very well have invented herself" (*New York Times* 22 Aug. 1971) 15.

5. Speaking of her own family in an interview with Anne Koenen, *Conversations with Toni Morrison Morrison* commented:

One of the characteristics of Black women's experiences was that they did not have to choose between a career and a home. They did both. . . . I know my mother and father, my grandmother and grandfather, and the people that lived around me, they thought they were doing something important. And I don't know if they "loved" each other or not, but they took careful care of one another and there was something clear and common about what they were doing . . . It had to do with raising children, with being morally coherent people. Maybe that's a boring little life, but it seemed to me that was what was strong about it. Because of the dual responsibility that Black women had—when they were left, they didn't collapse. They didn't have crutches in the first place, so with nothing but themselves to rely on they just had to carry on. And that, I think, is absolutely extraordinary and marvellous. (72)

In her 1979 commencement address at Barnard College, Morrison presents her young female audience with her vision of black womanhood:

I am suggesting that we pay as much attention to our nurturing sensibilities as to our ambition. You are moving in the direction of freedom and the function of self-fulfilment and the consequences of that fulfilment should be to discover that there is something just as important as your are. In your rainbow journey toward the realization of personal goals, don't make choices based only on your security and your safety. . . . Let your might and power emanate from the place in you that is nurturing and caring.

Quoted in Marilyn Sanders Mobley, "Narrative Dilemma: Jadine as Cultural Orphan in *Tar Baby*," *Toni Morrison: Critical Perspectives, Past and Present*, ed., Henry Louis Gates, Jr., and K. A. Appiah (New York: Amistad) 286.

6. "The One Out of Sequence" (1980), in *Conversations with Toni Morrison* 67-83.

7. In the interview with Koenen, *Conversations with Toni Morrison*, Morrison elaborates: "When I talked to a very young black girl recently, it seemed to me that she had never heard of anything. They've grown up like they never had grandmothers. Or if they had them, they never paid them any attention. Kill your ancestors, you kill all" (73).

8. "Rootedness: The Ancestor as Foundation," *Black Women Writers (1950-1980)*, ed. Mari Evans (New York: Doubleday, 1984) 344.

9. (1987) in *Conversations with Toni Morrison* 234-38.

10. (1983) in *Conversations with Toni Morrison* 138-55.

11. Toni Morrison, *The Bluest Eye* (New York: Washington Square, 1970). All subseqent quotations will be from this edition.

12. (160-161) "Text and Countertext in *The Bluest Eye*," *Toni Morrison*, ed. Henry Louis Gates, Jr., and K. A. Appiah (New York: Amistad, 1993).

13. "I was sitting back in my seat, and I had taken a big bite of that candy and it pulled a tooth right out of my mouth. I could have cried . . . I don't believe I ever got over that. There I was, five months pregnant, trying to look like Jean Harlow, and a front tooth gone. Everything went then" (98).

14. As quoted in Karen Carmean's *Toni Morrison's World of Fiction* 18. Richard O. Moore, dir., "The Writer in America," Perspective Films, 1978.

15. Toni Morrison, *Tar Baby* (New York: Plume 1981) 305. All subsequent quotations will be from this edition.

16. Interview with Judith Wilson (1981), *Conversations with Toni Morrison* 131.

17. (1985) *Conversations with Toni Morrison* 194.

18. Ibid.

19. *Conversations with Toni Morrison* 122.

Works Cited

Bassin, Donna, Margaret Honey, and Meryle Mahrer Kaplan, eds. *Representations of Motherhood*. New Haven: Yale UP, 1994.

Carmean, Karen. *Toni Morrison's World of Fiction*. Troy, New York: Whitston, 1993.

Christian, Barbara. *Black Feminist Criticism: Perspectives on Black Women Writers*. New York: Pergamon, 1985.

Cosslett, Tess. *Women Writing Childbirth: Modern Discourses of Motherhood*. Manchester, England: Manchester UP, 1994.

Davis, Cynthia A. "Self, Society, and Myth in Toni Morrison's Fiction." *Toni Morrison*. Ed. Harold Bloom. New York: Chelsea, 1990. 7-25.

Denard, Carolyn. "The Convergence of Feminism and Ethnicity in the Fiction of Toni Morrison." *Critical Essays on Toni Morrison*. Ed. Nellie Y. McKay. Boston: G. K. & Co., 1988.

Erickson, Peter. "Images of Nurturance in *Tar Baby*." *Toni Morrison: Critical Perspectives, Past and Present*. Ed. Henry Louis Gates, Jr., and K. A. Appiah. New York: Amistad, 1993. 293-307.

Gibson, Donald. "Text and Countertext in *The Bluest Eye*." *Toni Morrison: Critical Perspectives, Past and Present.* Ed. Henry Louis Gates and K. A. Appiah. New York: Amistad, 1993.

Harris, Trudier. *Fiction and Folklore: The Novels of Toni Morrison.* Knoxville: U of Tennessee P, 1991.

Holloway, Karla, and Stephanie Demetrakopoulos. *New Dimensions in Spirituality: A Biracial and Bicultural Reading.* New York: Greenwood, 1987.

Lowinsky, Naomi Ruth. *Stories from the Motherline: Reclaiming the Mother-Daughter Bond, Finding Our Feminine Souls.* Los Angeles: Jeremy P. Tarcher, 1992.

Luxton, Meg. *More Than a Labour of Love.* Toronto: Women's Educational Press, 1980.

Mobley, Marilyn Sanders. "Narrative Dilemmas: Jadine as Cultural Orphan in *Tar Baby*." *Toni Morrison: Critical Perspectives, Past and Present.* Ed. Henry Louis Gates, Jr., and K. A. Appiah. New York: Amistad, 1993. 284-92.

Morrison, Toni. *The Bluest Eye.* New York: Washington Square, 1970.

——. "Rootedness: The Ancestor as Foundation." *Black Women Writers: (1950-1980).* Ed. Mari Evans. New York: Doubleday, 1984. 339-45.

——. *Tar Baby.* New York: Plume, 1981.

——. "What the Black Woman Thinks About Women's Lib." *New York Times Magazine* 22 Aug. 1971: 15.

Pettis, Joyce. "Difficult Survival." *Sage* 4.2 (1987): 26-29.

Reyes, Angelita. "Ancient Properties in the New World: The Paradox of the 'Other' in Toni Morrison's *Toni Morrison*." *Black Scholar* 17 (1986): 19-25.

Samuels, Wilfred, and Clenora Hudson-Weems. *Toni Morrison.* Boston: Twayne, 1990.

Silverman, Kaja. *The Subject of Semiotics.* New York: Oxford UP, 1983.

Taylor-Guthrie, Danille. *Conversations with Toni Morrison.* Jackson: UP of Mississippi, 1994.

Traylor, Eleanor W. "The Fabulous World of Toni Morrison: *Tar Baby*." *Critical Essays on Toni Morrison.* Ed. Nellie Mckay. Boston: G. K. Hall, 1988. 135-49.

Willis, Susan. "Eruptions of Funk: Historicizing Toni Morrison." *Black Literature and Literary Theory.* Ed. Henry L. Gates, Jr. New York: Methuen, 1984. 263-83.

7

SEEDS OF SHAME OR SEEDS OF CHANGE?
WHEN DAUGHTERS GIVE BIRTH TO THEIR FATHERS' CHILDREN

Brenda Daly

She managed to scoop the baby into the mat and crawl to the phone and they came and got her, resting the child between her legs, the cord still strung between them . . . They had to keep her awake, she kept trying to die. ("In the name of Jesus Christ of Nazareth, might I have a drink of water?") she thought.
—Carolivia Herron, *Thereafter Johnnie*

Little is known about how incested daughters experience pregnancy and childbirth; in fact, incest and pregnancy/childbirth are usually treated as mutually exclusive topics. One explanation for this lacuna in feminist scholarship may be that, since few father-daughter incest narratives end in childbirth, researchers have simply not become aware of the problem of incestuous childbirths.[1] Yet another possibility is that, due to feminist preferences for psychological rather than biological definitions of father-daughter incest, attention has not been paid to biological aspects of incest, such as pregnancy and childbirth. Nevertheless, a growing number of father-daughter incest stories by women do end in childbirth, and these narratives deserve careful scrutiny. Why? My answer is that when contemporary women write father-daughter incest narratives, they suggest new ways of interpreting and resisting patriarchal definitions of pregnancy and childbirth. Consider, for example, the Biblical story of Lot. This paradigmatic story of father-daughter incest demonstrates that, under patriarchy, violation of the incest taboo will be tolerated if the act has a "higher" purpose: to preserve the father's seed. As Katz Rothman argues, in patriarchal societies "the essential concept is the 'seed'" (141), undoubtedly because whoever controls the seed controls the future. As a result of this focus, the Biblical tale of Lot tells us nothing about how he lost his wife or how his daughters experienced their pregnancies and childbirths. The tale was not theirs to tell.

Now that women are describing incest experiences, as well as experiences of pregnancy and childbirth, they are also offering new answers to the question: who controls the seed when daughters bear their fathers' children? Two recent novels by and about African American women, Sapphire's *Push* (1996) and Carolivia Herron's *Thereafter Johnnie* (1991) portray such pregnancies and childbirths while, significantly, when a pregnancy occurs in father-daughter incest novels by and about white women, they almost always end with abortions.[2] For example, in Joyce Carol Oates's *You Must Remember This* (1987), a working-class white daughter who has an incestuous relationship with a surrogate father (her uncle), has an abortion arranged and paid for by her uncle. By contrast, in Alice Walker's *The Color Purple* (1982), Celie, who is poor and black, gives birth to what she believes to be her biological father's children. One might conclude that Celie gives birth rather than aborting because she lacks access to medical information; however, as Alice Walker has pointed out, abortion has long been taboo in the African American community because, under slavery, children could so easily be taken from their birth parents.[3] This difference in racial history also helps to explain why, when the incestuous surgeon-father in *Thereafter Johnnie* tries to force his daughter Patricia to submit to an abortion, she resists. Like Lot's daughters, Patricia wishes to bear her father's child.

However, since incestuous pregnancies have been reported in white families of different social classes, it is important to at least ask why white women novelists rarely depict pregnancies resulting from incest since, in actuality, father-daughter incest does occur in middle- and upper-class white families.[4] In the 1950s, for example, the eldest daughter in the wealthy and socially prominent Van Derbur family was, she believes, impregnated by her father. This information became public years later, and then only because the youngest Van Derbur daughter, Marilyn, Miss America 1958, acknowledged that she was an incest survivor. As a result of this public admission in *People* magazine in 1991, the Van Derbur daughters become research subjects, and according to Lenore Terr: "While Gwendolyn Mitchell remembered the fact that she was abused, she apparently did not remember everything; for example, she does not remember penetration, though there is some reason to believe she was taken to an abortionist by her father" (quoted in Freyd 76). Assuming pregnancy did occur, Van Derbur was clearly more interested in protecting his "good" name than in protecting his seed. This preference for abortion by white fathers seems to prevail regardless of social class. For example, in *Peyton Place* (1956) Grace Metallious portrays a doctor who performs an abortion after learning that his patient has been impregnated by her working-class, alcoholic father.

Another example of an actual pregnancy resulting from incest, this time in a middle-class rural white family in Iowa, is reported by psychiatrist Christian Hageseth in *A Thirteen Moon Journal*. According to Hageseth, one of his female patients told him that she was born of incest and later incested by her own father/grandfather. Without using his patient's names, Hageseth explains, "The summer before coming into therapy . . . two older sisters took her aside and confided she was not actually their real sister. . . . She was conceived by her oldest sister, now deceased, and her father. Her mother (really grandmother) kept the secret, raising her as if her own child" (267-68). Apparently, the family's isolation made it possible for them to keep their shameful secret. This Iowa farm family recalls Smiley's *A Thousand Acres* (1991) which portrays father-daughter incest in a middle-class family without, however, even a hint that the father might impregnate his daughters. Instead, death and sterility—for the daughters, as for the land—are imagined as likely consequences of such a patriarchal violation. Since Smiley's main goal was to rewrite Shakespeare's *King Lear,* she emphasizes the psychological, as opposed to the physiological after-effects of incestuous violation, thereby providing her Goneril and Regan (Ginny and Rose) with plausible motives for cruelty toward their aging father. Smiley may also have understood that, while readers would tolerate a story of father-daughter incest in a middle-class white family, they would reject a novel that depicted graphic sex or what might be even more taboo: the birth of a child of incest.

Regardless of Smiley's intentions, her novel was clearly acceptable to many middle-class (mostly) white readers,[5] as may be inferred from the fact that *A Thousand Acres* won the Pulitzer Prize in 1992. By contrast, although highly praised by African American critics such as Barbara Christian and Gloria Naylor, *Thereafter Johnnie,* also published in 1991, has been ignored by most white readers and by literary critics. One reason may be that Smiley uses the familiar codes and conventions of realism, while Herron's novel is so complex that one critic describes her as the James Joyce of African American literature. But Herron's novel may also have been resisted because, unlike Smiley's, it not only portrays the act of father-daughter incest in highly erotic language, but depicts the birth of a child from this union. The child becomes a major character, as well as a major narrator of this complex, postmodern novel which shifts its temporal zone from the past to the present to the future, while also shifting linguistic registers from the divine to the mundane. However, even before the backlash against incest stories that began during the Reagan/Bush era, most readers were highly critical of women writers who gave detailed accounts of sexual violence. For example,

Oates's fiction has frequently been criticized as being "too violent," probably because she does not draw back from detailed depictions of sexual violence, including father-daughter incest. While it may be impossible to establish why white women writers omit graphic scenes of impregnation or childbirth, it must be noted that incested white daughters of all classes choose abortions, even when abortion is illegal—as, for example, in *Peyton Place* and *You Must Remember This,* both set in the 1950s.

By contrast, a welfare daughter in Sapphire's *Push* and an upper-middle-class daughter in Herron's *Thereafter Johnnie,* both set in the late twentieth century when abortions are legal, bear their fathers' children. However, each daughter, Sapphire's Precious and Herron's Patricia, offers different reasons for giving birth. After being raped repeatedly by her poor, crack-addicted father, Precious Jones, who cannot read or write, gives birth to two of her father's children. Conversely, after "seducing" her father, a wealthy surgeon, Patricia Snowdon, a student of "dead" languages at Howard University, becomes pregnant and insists on giving birth. Patricia refuses to allow her father to perform an abortion because she believes that, by giving birth to the child, she is, like Lot's daughters, living out an apocalyptic myth. Even though Patricia's father abandons her when she insists on bearing his child, he does provide generous financial support. Twelve-year-old, illiterate Precious, who is brutalized by both her unemployed parents, gives birth to her first child, a little "mongoloid" girl, because she doesn't know she has a choice; four years later, though still illiterate, she chooses to bear her father's child, a little boy, because she believes that abortion is morally wrong and because she yearns to love and be loved by the baby. Precious neither gives nor receives love from her first child because her own mother claims the infant as hers in order to collect more welfare money. In actuality, the child's maternal great-grandmother, who does not live with the mother or incested daughter, cares for the child that Precious calls "Little Mongo."

The linguistic registers in these novels also differ dramatically: *Thereafter Johnnie* shifts rapidly from epic rhetoric to the vernacular, while *Push* employs a language that one reviewer describes as "a hobbled, minimal English that defies the conventions of spelling and usage and dispenses with all verbal decorum" (Mahoney 9). While Herron's novel is a complex rewriting of Western myth and literature, *Push* might be defined as a contemporary slave/literacy narrative in which freedom is achieved, at least in part, through the protagonist's struggle to learn to read and write. However, even though pregnancy and childbirth are described primarily in naturalistic detail in *Push,* the novel's title refers not only to the physical act of giving birth, but also to the daughter/ mother's act of giving birth to herself, through language; in both activities Precious is encouraged to "push." As the novel closes, 18-year-old Precious, who has never had a boyfriend, describes childbirth and its after-effects in these words: "stretch marks and torn pussy from babies's head bust me open. That HURT. Hours hours push push push! Then he out, beautiful. Jus' a beautiful baby. But I'm not" (116). Even after Precious learns that her father infected her with the AIDS virus, she persists in her struggle to learn to read and write, continuing to "push" herself free from sexual slavery to her mother and father.

By contrast, Patricia chooses to bear her father's child because she believes the seed of their incestuous union will bring about an end to the United States, a nation conceived in patriarchal racism. Johnnie, the seed of Patricia's union with her father, is mute until age fourteen—a muteness that begins in infancy after she witnesses the last incestuous act. Johnnie begins to speak only after learning that she has a father, and, following her mother's suicide three years later, she begins a quest for the story of her origins, a questioning of each member of the Snowdon family. From her sister/aunt Eva, a lesbian whose rape by a stranger is structurally equivalent to Patricia's rape by/seduction of her father, Johnnie's conception is described in feminist, mythical terms: overhearing someone at the Black Cultural Center suggest, "Perhaps a black boy will be born in Harlem to raise the true black nation," Eva tells Johnnie, "No, I said, it will be a girl, and she won't be in Harlem, and she won't raise it, and the nation will not be true black" (98). From sister/aunt Cynthia Jane, who has become a nun, Johnnie learns that Patricia "believed in her myths, she actually quoted Lot's daughter to me, 'Come, let us make our father drink wine, and we will lie with him, that we may preserve seed of our father,' as if we lived at the end of the world" (207). Patricia herself, like a contemporary daughter of Lot, records her pursuit of her father in her journal: "I had to work so hard to get you to make love to me and I wanted so much to have a baby and so I got pregnant. But then you . . . wanted to give me an abortion" (31).

Despite significant differences, both novels depict daughters who struggle to act as agents of their own bodies even though their pregnancies and childbirths have already been defined by linguistic codes enforced through institutional power. As illustrated in these novels, the binary oppositions established by mythical narratives (god is to man as man is to woman) have shaped the beliefs and practices of religious, familial, legal, scientific, governmental and medical institutions and discourses, all of which exert control over women's lives and bodies. In obedience to mythical structures, patriarchal law defines children as the property of the father. As feminist critics have also noted, scientific language is often based on such binary oppositions: the language of reproductive technocrats—in which eggs are "harvested," for example—presumes the absence of the mother as a speaking, involved subject. Instead, as Gena Corea has shown, she is a "machine" whose role is that of passive object of scientific experimentation. Similarly, the language of so-called surrogacy contracts separates the mother not only from her child, but from her own uterus, her own body. In short, it is generally assumed that the seed is the property of the father who sows it in the body of a woman.

For this reason, when women tell their own stories of mothering, they find it necessary to resist and revise mythical structures that have, for centuries, shaped patriarchal narratives of motherhood. For example, although pregnancy and childbirth have long been regarded as instinctive activities, it is important to differentiate pregnancy and childbirth from the activity of child care, not only because a woman may choose to have an abortion or give her child up for adoption, but also because childbirth is, to some extent, an instinctive act, while competent child care requires a particular kind of thought.[6] Because the work of childcare is often considered "instinctive," feminist philosopher Sara Ruddick found it necessary to begin *Maternal Thinking* by persuading readers that mothers do, in fact, think. If child care is defined as an activity that requires a certain kind of thought—thinking concerned with the preservation, growth, and social acceptability of children—it would seem to follow that pregnancy and childbirth are instinctive activities. However, according to Tess Coslett, even this binary opposition—between instinctive childbirth and thoughtful child care—cannot withstand close scrutiny. According to Coslett, childbirth itself is not a completely instinctive activity. As she demonstrates in *Women Writing Childbirth,* a woman's experiences of pregnancy and childbirth may be affected by a range of often contradictory discourses that shape her attitudes toward and experiences of these life-altering events. To some extent, a woman's actual childbirth experience may depend on which stories she believes. Thus, whether a woman is single or married, white or black, she is likely to have expectations, even if unarticulated, about pregnancy and childbirth.

Although neither Ruddick nor Coslett examines the influence of incestuous conception on women's perceptions of pregnancy and childbirth, both offer insights useful for analyzing women's representations of such experiences. For example, according to Coslett, the belief that a woman can give birth without pain, the assumption of proponents of natural childbirth, is based on a racist concept, "the primitive woman." As

Coslett illustrates, the primitive woman is "often identified as African, she goes into the bushes on her own, gives birth painlessly and without fuss, and returns immediately to her work in the fields" (9). This primitive notion of childbirth is repudiated, Coslett shows, in Toni Morrison's *Beloved,* a novel that also provides a historical framework—the trauma of slavery—for analyzing differences in representations of incestuous pregnancies and childbirths in novels by and about African American women. The historical trauma, although not central in either *Push* or *Thereafter Johnnie,* frames both narratives, helping to explain why African American daughters claim the children of men, including fathers, for whom they have functioned as sexual slaves. In *Thereafter Johnnie,* the struggle for socio-linguistic control of the seed of women's bodies becomes even more complex when the incested daughter/mother chooses a lesbian partner, while in *Push* it is complicated by the fact that the mother is a twelve-year-old child who cannot read or write.

Pregnancy and Childbirth in Push

Precious Jones can claim the right to mother her child only after she achieves some freedom from her abusive parents, primarily through the support of teachers in a literacy program called "Each One, Teach One." As Precious is nurtured by Ms. Rain, who teaches her to read and write, she learns to claim her right to mother herself and her child. The novel is narrated by Precious, who begins with this oral self-presentation: "I was left back when I was twelve because I had a baby for my fahver. That was in 1983. I was out of school for a year. This gonna be my second baby" (3). At the time her first child was born, Precious had no way to resist the abuse of her parents, both of whom treated her as a slave—an object of property. However, four years later, when Precious is sixteen and in the ninth grade, she begins to resist injustice. She explains, "I got suspended from school 'cause I'm pregnant which I don't think is fair. I ain' did nothin'!" Precious, who stands over five feet nine inches tall and weighs over 200 pounds, defends herself by physically attacking the white woman who suspends her. At this stage, she is not capable of finding words to defend herself. However, the suspension proves fortuitous because, once sent to an alternative school, Precious is encouraged to "push" to learn, just as a kind attendant had urged her to push to give birth to her first child.

In contrast to this kind attendant, who treats Precious as a "you," her parents view her as an "it," a creature born only to serve their needs. For example, in one of the novel's many shocking moments, twelve-year-old Precious experiences her first labor pains while being severely beaten by her mother:

Ahh wump! I never felt no shit like that before. Sweat was breaking out on my forehead, pain like fire was eating me up. I jus' standing there 'n pain hit me, then pain go sit down, then pain git up 'n hit me harder! 'N she standing there screaming at me, "Slut! Goddam slut! You fuckin' cow! . . . ." Pain hit me again, then she hit me. I'm on the floor groaning, "Mommy please, Mommy please, please Mommy! Mommy! Mommy! MOMMY! Then she KICK me side of my face! (10)

Finally, when a neighbor calls 911, Precious is released from her mother's abuse. Lying in a "ball from [the] pain," of her mother's beating mingled with the pain of labor, Precious experiences the kindness of a "Spanish guy in EMS uniform" who, as he touches her forehead and belly, asks, "What's your name?" Addressing her by name, he counsels, "Precious, it's almost here. I want you to push, you hear me momi, when that shit hit you again, go with it and push, Preshecita. *Push*" (10). Four years later, pregnant again, Precious dreams of riding an elevator to the alternative school on the nineteenth floor. As the elevator door opens, she sees the "coffee-cream-colored man from Spanish talk land," and he says, "Push, Precious, you gonna hafta push" (17). Based on this I/thou experience, Precious becomes aware of her humanity.

As a result of this and other similar experiences, Precious transforms the painful experience of childbirth into a metaphor for her own birth: heroically, she pushes to acquire the language skills that will enable her to survive economically while mothering her second child. Yet even before Precious acquires linguistic competence, her consciousness—as well as her experiences—are shaped by a range of institutional discourses: politics, education, social services, religion. For example, in her bedroom, Precious has hung a picture of Louis Farrakhan which bears the caption, "THE BLACK MAN'S TIME" (24). Because she cannot read, Precious doesn't notice that Farrakhan does not identify a time for black women. However, Precious is aware of the power of language, particularly when used by institutions that control her life. She is angry, for example, that her school has sent her file to the alternative school; however, because she cannot read, she cannot protest what might be false information. Precious believes that "every time they wants to fuck with her or decide her life—here they come with the mutherfucking file" (30). She also knows that both she and her first child are defined, according to welfare files, as her mother's dependents, an arrangement financially beneficial to her mother but which keeps Precious dependent on her. Precious also knows that G.E.D. tests define her as lacking in basic math and reading skills—"The tesses paint a picture of me wif no brain" (33)—despite the fact that her math teacher identifies her as a good student. The tests, Precious observes, render her "invisible."

Although Precious is illiterate, she recognizes that these official discourses define reality; moreover, she understands that these monologic discourses deny her a voice. When Precious becomes a student at the alternative school, she learns a different kind of language, a dialogic language: after attentively reading what Precious writes, the teacher asks questions that stimulate her pupil to think for herself. Like the medical attendant who encourages Precious to push with her body, Ms. Rain encourages Precious to push with words: "Write what's on your mind, push yourself to see the letters that represent the words you're thinking" (62-63). When Precious writes, "li Mg o mi m," the teacher translates, "Little Mongo on my mind" (63). Then the teacher writes the question, "Who is Little Mongo?" (63). In this way, Precious gives birth to herself through language, learning how to care for herself and her unborn child. As Coslett points out, the discourses of natural childbirth and medicine may affect childbirth experiences of middle-class women, but Precious is so young and poor that she has not had access to either discourse. When her first child was born, Precious had never heard of prenatal care. However, during her second pregnancy, Precious knows how babies are made, and after the birth of her child, she understands what her father has done to her: "I think I was rape" (70), she says.

Although confused about feeling some pleasure during intercourse—"I HATE myself when I feel good" (60)—she tries to forget that during her second pregnancy when she says, "I got a baby in me" (59). She also recognizes that she "hated borning the first one. No fun. Hurt. Now again" (59). Part of the confusion comes from the fact that, having been sexually violated by both parents, she has no clear sense of her own desires or even her own body. Precious wonders, "Why can't I see myself, feel when I end and begin?" (34). Through language, especially through dialogues with Miss Rain, Precious begins to claim her identity—her body, mind, and emotions. As a result, she says, "I don't pretend I'm not pregnant no more. I let it above my neck, in my head" (64). In these words, Precious defines her pregnancy as both a body/mind experience, not as a strictly physical or instinctive event. She recalls that, following the birth of Little Mongo, the pain from "the bloody tear between her legs, the black-blue on the side where her mother had kicked her" were even worse than the pain of father-rape: "Even her father who came to her in the night had not held her but had pushed her back and flung his pee-pee smelling thing in her mouth, then her vagina" (18). Despite these painful memories, the now sixteen-year-old Precious, who is seven months pregnant, decides to keep her second child: "I know too who I'm pregnant for. But I can't change that. Abortion is a sin. I hate bitches who kill their babies. They should kill them, see how they like it!" (65).

Readers are not told where Precious has learned that "abortion is a sin," nor is it clear whether anti-abortion discourse, rather than only her own desires, influence her choice to keep her child. We do know, however, that Precious identifies with the unborn child: because she wishes to be valued, to be precious, she is determined to value her unborn child. She wants the child to learn to read and to think of its mother as smart. Precious also wants to claim this child as her own, something she had been denied with her first child: "This is my baby. My muver took little Mongo but she ain' taking this one. I am comp'tant" (66). Precious understands that, to claim her independence from her parents, she must demand official recognition that this child is hers. The danger is that if Precious assumes, as do many parents in a capitalistic society, that children are defined as property, she may also assume it is her right to abuse that property. Slave owners held such views, as Morrison reminds us in *Beloved*. However, as Precious is nurtured in school, and as her ability to write is nurtured, she begins to think of her child, not as property, but as an entity with a consciousness separate from her own. Just as Ms. Rain talks to Precious, asking questions and responding in writing in her journal, Precious begins to write to her child to teach him or her the ABCs. "Listen baby," she writes:

> A is fr Afrc
>> (for Africa)
> B is for u bae
>> (you baby)
> C is cl w bk
>> (colored we black)
> D is dog
> E is el l/m
>> (evil like mama)
> F is Fuck (67)
> And on, through the entire 26 letters of the alphabet.

With the help of Ms. Rain, Precious is learning to value herself, to establish boundaries, to express her needs and desires, and, through the example of nurturant teaching, to mother herself. Precious recognizes that her mother, along with a racist culture, has failed to protect her from abuse: "She ain' come in here and say, Carl Kenwood Jones—that wrong! Git off Precious like that! Can't you see Precious is a beautiful chile like white chile in magazines or on toilet paper wrappers. Precious is a blue-eyed skinny chile whose hair is long braids, long long braids" (66). Precious has been defined as a person without value by official and familial discourses, as well as by what Carmen Luke calls the pedagogies of popular culture. However, at the alternative school, Precious is learning alternative ways of thinking about herself and her child. She learns, for example, that women can be heroes. That is why, after hearing from Ms. Rain that Harriet Tubman "leaded over 300 people out of slavery" (65), Precious places a poster of Harriet next to Farrakhan's, and she listens when her teacher describes Farrakhan as an "antiSemitic, homophobic fool" (76). Ms. Rain also challenges the homophobia expressed by her female students by coming out as a lesbian. Ms. Rain values herself and, as Precious becomes a more competent reader and writer—reading Ann Petry and Langston Hughes, for example—she learns that she too has a right to value herself.

Although childbirth is usually regarded as an interruption in one's education, Precious transforms it into a meaningful chapter in her schooling. For example, she names her second child, Abdul Jamal Louis Jones, explaining that "Abdul" means "servant of god," and Louis is for "Farrakhan" (69). The pain of childbirth also prompts Precious to reflect on the relationship between the history of slavery and her own rape: "What my fahver do is what Farrakhan said the white man did to the black woman. Oh it was terrible and he dood it in front of the black man; that's really terrible. . . . This spozed to hurt the black man even more than it hurt the woman getting rape—for the black man to have to see this raping" (70). As Precious struggles to survive following Abdul's birth, her experiences become an ironic commentary on the notion that the black man felt greater pain than the black woman. For example, because Precious claims both Abdul and Little Mongo as her own when interviewed by a welfare official, her mother loses welfare income. Angry at this loss, Precious's mother beats her when she returns from the hospital, forcing the young mother to seek shelter elsewhere. Homeless and still recovering from Abdul's birth, Precious nevertheless refuses to give up her child. The kindly Ms. Rain had warned, "If you keep Abdul you might have nothing" (72) and had suggested, "Being a good mother might mean letting your baby be raised by someone who is better able than you to meet the child's needs" (74). But Precious asserts her own point of view: "I is be bt meet cldls ed," which Miss Rain translates: "(I is best able to meet my child's need.)" (74).

This statement becomes questionable in light of events following Precious's release from the hospital: homeless, she returns to the hospital where a nurse who doesn't know her, but who does know she is still bleeding, refuses to allow her to return to the maternity ward. During a night in a cold armory, Precious is so weak that she cannot prevent her child's blanket from being stolen. She says, "my pussy feels torn apart, my lower back pain me, my bresses leaking milk" (79). Given the fact that her survival is threatened, it is important to ask, yet again, why Precious insists on assuming the burden of caring for Abdul. Is she simply responding "instinctively" to a child that has suckled at her breast? Has she been influenced by her grandmother who says, "Onle dog dro babee an wak off" which Ms. Rain translates, "(only a dog will drop a baby and walk off)" (73). Ms. Rain also asks, "Where was you grandmother when your father was abusing you?" and "What is going to be the best thing for you in this situation?" (73). The important point is that, even though Ms. Rain questions whether Precious has the capacity to care for a child, she respects her pupil's humanity; therefore, she does not try to force her to give up her child. Ms. Rain may well wonder whether Precious is over-identifying with her child, thereby jeopardizing his well-being along with her own; however, she does not try to override the young mother's judgment.

Ironically, Ms. Rain's maternal teaching methods have had a powerful influence on Precious's choice: having learned to value herself through Ms. Rain's dialogic use of language, Precious establishes a similar bond with her unborn child. Since this bond is already established by the time Abdul is born, it may be that Precious, though still a child herself, actually is the person best able to meet the needs of her child. Certainly her desire is strong; she risks her life to care for Abdul, and she "pushes" herself to achieve test scores in math and English that identify her as someone with employable skills. Through her resistance to a racist and sexist society, particularly her insistence on the right to both education and motherhood, Precious asks readers to question a society that assumes that education and childbirth are mutually exclusive activities. Precious also asks readers to examine the values of a society that not only tolerates the abuse of children but punishes the victim rather than the perpetrator. "Why no one put Carl in jail after I have a baby by him when I'm twelve?" she asks; "Is it my fault because I didn't talk to polices?" (127). But how is a child of twelve to know that she should report this heinous act to the police?

I would argue, then, that the second time Precious experiences pregnancy and childbirth, she suffers physical pain similar to her first; however, her psychic pain is far different, primarily because, though not yet fully literate, she has begun to assert her own reality. Precious has learned a dialogic literacy that enables her to claim her own perspective while, at the same time, valuing other points of view. After a brief stay in the home of the Dream Keeper, the Langston Hughes House, Precious finds a long-term place in Advancement House, which provides child care that will allow her to return to school. As Precious gains greater competency in reading, she also learns to question what she reads. For example, when Ms. Rain assigns Alice Walker's *The Color Purple,* she learns that "a group of black men wanted to stop movie from the book. Say unfair picture of nigger men. She ax me what do I think? Unfair picture? Unfortunately it a picture I know" (85). When Ms. Rain also says that *The Color Purple* has been criticized for its "fairy tale ending," Precious defends the novel even though, unlike Walker's Celie, who learns that her father really wasn't her biological father, Precious knows that her biological father not only raped her, but also infected her with the AIDS virus. Asked to write her life story, Precious begins, "A boy come out my pussy. Was nothing. A dark spot in the sky; then turn life in me" (97). When she stops writing, feeling "my blood a giant river swell up inside me and I'm drowning. . . . Feel like a giant river I never cross in front me now," Ms. Rain urges, "You can't stop now, Precious, you gotta push" (99).

Pregnancy and Childbirth in Thereafter Johnnie

Language is not everything, yet to some degree the experiences of pregnancy and childbirth are shaped by male-dominated discourses through which men engage in a struggle for social control of women's bodies and the seed of their labor. This struggle for symbolic control assumes mythical proportions in *Thereafter Johnnie,* the story of incest in an upper-middle-class African American family in Washington, D.C. The novel is an "epic achievement," as Barbara Christian declares, with an epic structure "composed of 24 parts like Homer's *Odyssey* and like it demonstrates that *sex* is *religion* is *nation,* that, to use a Freudian term, 'family romance,' is a nation's soul" ("Epic Achievement" 6). The second daughter, Patricia, is depicted as coldly destroying her family— her mother, Camille, and her sisters, Cynthia Jane and Eva—in order to possess her father, John Christopher, and bear his child. Patricia violently rejects an abortion which John Christopher, a surgeon, wants to perform; instead she chooses to give birth to the child of their incestuous union, a daughter whom she calls "Johnnie." Some feminists may object to Herron's characterization of Patricia; nevertheless, the novel might be described as a feminist re-telling of the Biblical story of Lot, of a father seduced by his daughters. At the same time, Herron dramatizes father-daughter incest as the curse of slavery, but in the Snowdon family's fulfillment of the curse, as in the story of Lot, they engender the seed of a new nation.

Patricia's complicity in the incestuous relationship marks Herron's novel as a significant departure from those of Walker and Morrison, as Christian points out in her review: "Herron figures different forms of incest, sister/sister, father/daughter, almost as emblems of different mythic structures. But she does not present father-daughter incest, as Alice Walker does in *The Color Purple,* as a powerful father-figure's brutal assault upon a helpless girl-child, or as Toni Morrison does in *The Bluest Eye,* as a powerless father's sense that sexual love is all he can give his wounded daughter" ("Epic Achievement" 6). Because Patricia chooses to act the part of Lot's daughter, she plays a powerful role: creating and preserving the seed of a new nation. While problematizing the search for origins, the novel dramatizes the fulfillment of certain destructive patriarchal myths, implying that these actions eventually lead to the founding of a life-enhancing country of whose origins Johnnie and her descendants sing. Since John Christopher also seems to be reenacting a curse—the curse of slavery—Herron may actually intend the act of sexual intercourse between father and daughter to be interpreted as divine love, as *agape.* It is difficult to determine who initiated the incest. Did John Christopher begin to fondle his daughter at the age of two? If so, did his actions actually create the adult Patricia who appears to seduce her father? Or is the adult Patricia created by her own desire to live out the incest plot in patriarchal myths? On this point, the novel is deliberately ambiguous.[7]

Any analysis of *Thereafter Johnnie,* a highly complex novel, must take into account its representations of pregnancy and childbirth, its allusions to myths, as well as its structure—its parallel chapters, its beginning and ending, and its multiple points of view. Herron's depiction of Johnnie's birth is a good example of her ability both to fulfill and transform myths: the child is born of an incestuous union, signifying the destruction of a patriarchal family/nation, but she also becomes the child of a lesbian named Diotima, an "othermother" (to use Patricia Collins' term) who, after nurturing both Johnnie and her mother Patricia, founds a new nation. Johnnie tells us, "When I was held within my mother's body Diotima had been kind" (24). Because the narrative is so complex, only a second reading is likely to reveal that Johnnie's birth, portrayed as her mother Patricia's crucifixion, is cast as a "mythical" second coming. Likewise, only a second reading of the novel reveals the significance of the father/grandfather's initials, J. C., and his name, John Christopher. Named after two Biblical heroes, John and Christ, his role is to announce the coming of a (second) Christ, as did the Biblical John, and, historically, to come before Johnnie, as Christ came before her. These New Testament roles are linked to the Old Testament Lot whose seed, planted in his daughters, became the origins of a new family/nation. Patricia bears the seeds of a new nation established by Diotima and others who wish to nurture rather than destroy the planet.

As Christian notes, "As in the stories of the old gods (Zeus, Jehovah), incest is central to this contemporary family/national romance" ("Epic Achievement" 6), and Patricia's incestuous pregnancy is described as a re-enactment of an epic event: "There were two nations fighting in a single womb, each striving to kill the other, they came to America, and fell as one into sleep, dream, nightmare, upon the Potomac River. They shall awaken into death" (173). Patricia, who gives birth to Johnnie alone in her apartment bathroom, describes the pain of reliving this mythological conflict as "an orgasm that could not release itself" (134). The orgasm seems to release itself not with Johnnie's birth, but at Patricia's death which occurs when Johnnie reaches the age of 17 (the same age at which Patricia gave birth to Johnnie). Echoes of the crucifixion of Christ can be heard when, during Patricia's hospital stay following Johnnie's birth, she repeatedly calls for water, and for her mother, as if suffering on the cross of childbirth in the context of patriarchal history. Years after her actual birth, Johnnie also employs the language of childbirth to describe her mother's suicide: "It has been over ten years since her mother stepped into the Potomac. She does not want to think about it anymore. She thinks about it. Dilation and Cutterage" (169). Having been rendered mute after observing sexual intercourse between her mother and father/grandfather, Johnnie's first words, when she finally speaks fourteen years later, are "Daddy, Daddy!" (144), and when she writes, she repeats, "I HATE YOU MOMMY" (146). It is this Symbolic (mythical) language of mother-hatred, a binary system that enforces I/it hierarchical relationships, that Herron is resisting and rewriting in *Thereafter Johnnie.*

Birth into language, into the Symbolic, appears to necessitate an often unconscious fear and hatred of the mother, along with an overidealized love of the father. However, as Johnnie learns the stories of her conception and birth from her sister/aunts and mother/grandmother, she begins to hear and speak a more complex language. The story of Johnnie's birth is told, for example, through familial dialogues, as well as through a range of contending discourses. From her lesbian aunt Eva, Johnnie learns that her surgeon father/grandfather, John Christopher, had been jealous of the pleasure his three daughters shared in poetry. A chapter called "Three Witches," depicts the Snowdon daughters as "touching and playing in the snow like three maniacs, three witches, three weird sisters" (46) and again as "three Furies, three Graces, three Fates" (51). Johnnie observes, echoing the language of Shakespeare's

Macbeth, "They excluded you. They didn't want you or need you. When will they meet again? Your three daughters? When will those three meet again. Never, never again. Not since my mother stepped out above the Potomac River. . . . Not in thunder, lightning, or rain. But in snow" (53-54).[8] Threatened and excluded by his daughters' intimacy, "The King of Hearts" displays his power to remove and replace a dog's heart. "Do you want to learn to believe in life?" John Christopher commands:

Watch. A golden bird you say. A sick rose. A forbidden apple. Poetry. Yeats. Blake. Milton. That's all you talk about. It took blood and a flesh heart to imagine the golden bird to interpret the sick rose to envision the fruit. I will sew the blood and flesh heart back into the dog. Your poets are made of the blood and mire that you hate. (58)

Out of this desire to control conception, childbirth becomes for this father the site of a socio-linguistic struggle, not only among men of different races, but also between the discourses of poetry and science. Life, according to John Christopher, is enacted through scientific miracles, not through the sounds and rhythms of poetry. Up to this point, Patricia has avoided science and technology, preferring the study of poetry, but she is seduced by her father's display of scientific prowess, his "surgical magic" (54). Seeing the dog lying helpless, in the shape of an X— "spread-eagle on the operating table" (59)—Patricia decides to become her father's "bitch." She turns away from the circle of her sisters, the circle of poetry that threatens John Christopher. Eva says of her sisters, "When they first learned to read I was the one who led them toward the chapters of their desire" (111), but her sisters do not follow her lead, undoubtedly because the chapters of their early desire have been distorted by patriarchal images of women-bonding, such as Shakespeare's image of the three witches in Macbeth. John Christopher wants to usurp the power of life and death, of womb and tomb, that women "control" through childbirth. Science, then, is represented as a discourse of patriarchal control, the means by which John Christopher imagines that, like a contemporary Frankenstein, he manipulates birth and death.

When Patricia insists upon bearing her father's child, John Christopher learns the limits of patriarchal and scientific power. Herron portrays the sadomasochistic Snowdon father and daughter as re-enacting, not a "private" drama, but the historical trauma of slavery. To link father-daughter incest to the historical-psychological trauma of slavery, Herron employs a recurring letter "X." As in the scene in which John Christopher removes and restores a dog's heart, the letter X (it) calls attention to sexual slavery in its various guises. For example, the letter X appears in the rape of the slave Laetitia, one of Camille Snowdon's foremothers: "The young master between her legs with his hands gripped around her thighs, the old master at her head, his hands hooked under her shoulders and Laetitia was held in the air in the shape of an X in order to be fornicated" (238). The "X" surfaces again during John Christopher's courtship of Camille and, later, in his rape of their daughter, Patricia. Camille recalls that when Patricia was two, she acted "as if she had been struck by lightning. . . . I couldn't bend her arms and legs at all and when I picked her up she went into an X shape" (180). As if the traumatic memory of slavery is stored in their muscles, the Snowdons repeatedly reenact its torture.[9] Both John Christopher and Patricia appear to be addicted to their sexual enslavement.

The Snowdons enact, in mircrocosm, the patriarchal myths and discourses that lead to a struggle for global control that results, as readers understand only in retrospect, in the destruction of the United States. Only because Johnnie insists on learning and telling the various stories of her conception does this compulsion to repeat history come to an end. Hence, Johnnie's birth signifies both an end to a patriarchal nation and the beginning of another. This new nation, though of woman born, is fulfilled through a re-visioning of Biblical prophecy. According to the Book of Revelations, a war in heaven will follow the birth of a "man child": "A woman clothed with the sun, and the moon under her feet, and upon her head a crown of twelve stars. And she being with child cried, travailing in birth, and pained to be delivered" (12). However, in *Thereafter Johnnie,* Johnnie is a female child—"a tar baby warm and fat, looking out on the world with clear white-blue eyes" (133)—whose coming leads to war, not in heaven but on earth. Named Kristen Dolores at birth, which means " 'she before whom Christ sorrowed,' that is to say, Johnnie" (133), the "chiaroscuro" child is portrayed as the second coming prophesied in Revelations. Among the survivors of the apocalypse that destroys Washington, D.C., among those who find safety in a mountainous region in Mexico, are Johnnie's grandmother Camille and her othermother Diotima.

How does this nation differ from what has gone before? We are given only sketchy details. For example, we learn that Camille uses her scientific knowledge to ensure the group's survival rather than, like her husband, to achieve godlike power. Camille tells Johnnie, "A lot of the things I learned in order to teach science come in handy now. We've put everything we know together so we can grow decent vegetables and we know how to make clothes from animals and plants. It's not so bad, and we have one whole group interested in weaving" (177-78). The nation's first story teller is Diotima, a lesbian who bears the name of Plato's philosopher queen:

And I, Diotima, learned this tale from Diotima, the one who long ago came to us from the north where she knew the black maiden, who is Johnnie, Diotima came here to Puerto Escondido telling this tale and creating the storytelling tribe of Diotima so that we may know what has passed in the north and where there is such great silence there. (241)

Within the novel's complex time-frame, Patricia represents the present (already past) while Johnnie represents the future (already present), and Diotima's descendants represent the future of that future. But most important, history is told and retold to affirm the values of a matrilineal, democratic society. Heterosexism, portrayed as a form of sexual slavery, has apparently come to an end. Johnnie, who survives the destruction of Washington, D.C., becomes a bard who sings an "ancient song" (6) of her own conception: "And god said to Patricia, 'your moment is ended. Before this birth all the ages of your people have longed for you, but from the moment the child is born, thereafter Johnnie is the soul of your nation.' And so it was I was born once upon a time" (133). And so it is that Johnnie, the seed of shame, becomes a seed—and a voice—of cultural transformation.

In *Push* and *Thereafter Johnnie,* Sapphire and Herron portray the conceptions and births of incestuously conceived children in markedly different linguistic registers; however, both strive to resist and even to rewrite those discourses that, through the power of institutions, perpetuate racism, sexism, classism, and homophobia. The imaginative power of these novels is remarkable; unfortunately, it is for this very reason they are likely to offend many readers. Influenced by the current backlash against incest stories, some may refuse even to read these novels, while those who do read them will undoubtedly find much to criticize. Unaware of their own class and racial biases, some readers may be repulsed by the graphic manner in which Sapphire portrays child sexual abuse and childbirth; others may condemn Precious for using "crude" terms such as "pussy" to describe her anatomy. Some traditional Christian readers are likely to criticize Herron for rewriting the Biblical story of Lot. Finally, as Barbara Christian suggests, some feminists may object to Herron's depiction of Patricia, a daughter who initiates sex with her father in order to bear his child. These novels remind us, then, that there is no neutral ground from which—and no neutral language in which—to portray pregnancy and childbirth. These commonplace and miraculous processes are, in fact, deeply embedded in the Symbolic, the mythical language in which our pasts have been written and from which our futures are struggling to be born.

Notes

1. As early as the nineteenth century, women writers such as Mary Shelley violated the taboo against speaking out against father-daughter incest. For other examples, see Karen Jacoben McLennan's *Nature's Ban: Women's Incest Literature* (Northeastern UP, 1996), which includes women's incest narratives dating from the twelfth century to the early 1990s. Since the second wave of the women's movement, this canon has expanded rapidly to include, in addition to narratives mentioned in the body of this essay, Joyce Carol Oates's *A Garden of Earthly Delights* (Vanguard, 1966), Gayl Jones's *Corregidora* (1975; Rpt. Beacon P, 1986), Alice Walker's *The Color Purple* (Harcourt Brace Jovanovich, 1982), Toni Morrison's *Beloved* (Knopf, 1987); Buchi Emecheta's *The Family* (Braziller, 1990) and *Gwendolen* (Flamingo, 1990), Jane Smiley's *A Thousand Acres* (Knopf, 1991), Dorothy Allison's *Bastard Out of Carolina* (Penguin, 1992), Margaret Atwood's *The Robber Bride* (Bantam, 1993), Marilyn French's *Our Father* (Ballantine, 1994), Sally Patterson *Tubach's Memoirs of a Terrorist* (State University of New York Press, 1996), and many others. Many memoirs exposing father-daughter incest have also been written since the sixties: one of the best known is Maya Angelou's *I Know Why the Caged Bird Sings* (Random House, 1970); one of the earliest collections edited by Toni A. H. McNaron and Yarrow Morgan; *Voices in the Night: Women Speaking About Incest* (Pittsburgh, PA: Cleis P, 1982); and one of the most recent and controversial, Kathryn Harrison's *The Kiss* (Random House, 1997).

2. In *A Garden of Earthly Delights* (1966), Joyce Carol Oates portrays a migrant worker's daughter, Rosalie, who bears her father's child; however, we do not hear from Rosalie herself, a minor character in the novel. For a more complete analysis of father-daughter incest in this and other novels by Oates, see my *Lavish Self-Divisons: The Novels of Joyce Carol Oates* (Jackson: U of Mississippi, P, 1996).

3. In a video-taped interview, Alice Walker describes her own abortion as painful decision to break this taboo (Lannan Foundation, 5401 McConnell Ave., Los Angeles, CA 900666-7027).

4. This omission perpetuates racial and class stereotypes, as Melba Wilson argues (66, 130). Ralph Ellison makes a similar argument in *Invisible Man* (1952; Rpt. Vintage P, 1990).

5. Nevertheless, as I point out in *Authoring a Life: A Women's Survival in and through Literary Studies* (New York: State University of New York Press, 1998), Smiley's novel has been subjected to censorship. Also see Marina Leslie's "Incest, Incorporation, and *King Lear* in Jane Smiley's *A Thousand Acres*," *College English* 60.1 (Jan. 1998): 31-50.

6. I make this argument, along with my co-editor, Maureen T. Reddy, in the introduction to *Narrating Mothers: Theorizing Maternal Subjectivities* (Knoxville: U of Tennessee P, 1991).

7. I address this question more fully in an earlier essay, "Whose Daughter Is Johnnie? Revisionary Myth-making in Carolivia Herron's *Thereafter Johnnie*" in *Callaloo: A Journal of African American and African Arts and Letters* 18.2 (1995): 473-91.

8. Herron, who dedicates her novel, "For Sister Pamela Ann Smith, Janice Schuh Okulski, and The Villa Nova," identifies with the witch-sisters when she adds, "When Shall We Three Meet Again?" In 1992, Herron, who identifies as a lesbian, told Melba Wilson that she was abused at the age of three by a male relative and that "she wakes up every morning to a note pinned to her bed. . . . which says, 'Remember not to kill yourself today'" (Wilson 179).

9. Shoshana Felman argues that traumatic historical events "tend to repeat themselves . . . because their impact—as a consequence of trauma—takes effect and truly registers in history only through the gap of their traumatic repetition" (744). See her "Forms of Judicial Blindness, or the Evidence of What Cannot Be Seen: Traumatic Narratives and Legal Repetitions in the O. J. Simpson Case and in Tolstoy's *The Kretuzer Sonata*," *Critical Inquiry* 23 (Summer 1997): 738-88.

Works Cited

Arundell, Terry. *Mothers and Divorce: Legal, Economic, and Social Dilemmas.* Berkeley: U of California P, 1986.

Belenky, Mary Field, Blythe McVicker Clinchy, Nancy Rule Goldberger, and Jill Mattuck Tarule. *Women's Ways of Knowing: The Development of Self, Voice, and Mind.* New York: Basic, 1986.

Brownmiller, Susan. "Introduction." *The Best Kept Secret: Sexual Abuse of Children.* By Florence Rush. New York: McGraw-Hill, 1980. viii-ix.

Christian, Barbara. "Epic Achievement." Rev. of *Thereafter Johnnie. Women's Review of Books* 9.1 (Oct. 1991): 6-7.

Collins, Patricia Hill. "The Meaning of Motherhood in Black Culture and Black Mother-Daughter Relationships." *Sage* 4.2 (1987): 3-10.

Corea, Gena. *The Mother Machine.* New York: Harper and Row, 1985.

Coslett, Tess. *Women Writing Childbirth: Modern Discourses of Motherhood.* New York: Manchester UP, 1994.

Hageseth, Christian, III, M.D. *A Thirteen Moon Journal: A Psychiatrist's Journey Toward Inner Peace.* Fort Collins, CO: Berwick, 1991.

Herman, Judith Lewis, with Lisa Hirschman. *Father-Daughter Incest.* Cambridge, MA: Harvard UP, 1981.

Luke, Carmen, ed. *Feminisms and Pedagogies of Everyday Life.* Albany: State U of New York P, 1996.

Mahoney, Rosemary. "'Don't Nobody Want Me. Don't Nobody Need Me.'" Review of *Push* by Sapphire. *New York Times* Book Review (7 July 1996): 9.

Metalious, Grace. *Peyton Place.* New York: Simon & Schuster, 1956.

Morrison, Toni. *The Bluest Eye.* New York: Pocket, 1970.

Oates, Joyce Carol. *You Must Remember This.* New York: Dutton, 1987.

Rothman, Barbara Katz. "Beyond Mothers and Fathers: Ideology in a Patriarchal Society." *Mothering: Ideology, Experience, and Agency.* Ed. Evelyn Nakano Glenn, Grace Chang, Linda Rennie Forcey. New York: Routledge, 1994.

Ruddick, Sara. *Maternal Thinking: Toward a Politics of Peace.* Boston: Beacon, 1989.

Sapphire. *Push.* New York: Knopf, 1996.

Smiley, Jane. *A Thousand Acres.* New York: Knopf, 1991.

Terr, Lenore C. *Too Scared to Cry: Psychic Trauma in Childhood.* New York: Harper and Row, 1990.

Van Derbur, Marilyn. "The Darkest Secret." *People* 10 June 1991: 88-94.

Wilson, Melba. *Crossing the Boundary: Black Women Survive Incest.* London: Virago, 1993.

8

"INTO THE BIRTH HOUSE" WITH LOUISE ERDRICH

Julie Tharp

> When they were wild
> When they were not yet human
> When they could have been anything,
> I was on the other side ready with milk to lure them,
> And their father, too, each name a net in his hands.
>> "Birth," from *Baptism of Desire*

Louise Erdrich in her prolonged meditation on pregnancy and child-birth, *The Blue Jay's Dance: A Birth Year,* imagines women writers working together now to create an " intellectual quilt" (145). This "intellectual quilt" will provide the strength and vision of mothers who have written almost nothing until the last two decades; this maternal literature will offer gentleness but also tough endurance, survival. One of Erdrich's rich contributions to the quilt is her use of birth stories that celebrate survival within perilous conditions. This essay is focused on the function of those birth narratives in the novels *Love Medicine, Tracks, The Beet Queen,* and *Tales of Burning Love.* These four novels and a fifth, *Bingo Palace,* revolve around a cast of about two dozen characters, all of whom are interrelated by blood, marriage, and circumstance.[1] The birth stories told within the novels strike right at the heart of that inter-relationship, bringing not just biological families together, but connecting a variety of people over time, space, and differences of all kinds in a matrix that can leave no one adrift. While Erdrich does not dwell on the mother's perspective per se, her novels provide a maternal sensibility that is easily read through the birth stories.

All but one of Erdrich's fictional birth stories share an external point of view. No female character, with the exception of Pauline, relates her own delivery. While this would seem to be a problem if we are most interested in learning about the experience of childbirth from the mother's perspective, Erdrich's own comments offer a perfectly good explanation:

The person who experiences birth with the closest degree of awareness is the mother—but not only am I physically programmed to forget the experience to some degree . . . , I am overwhelmed by what is happening to me. I certainly can't take notes, jot down my sensations, or even have them with any perspective after a while. And then, once our baby is actually born, the experience of labor, even at its most intense, is eclipsed by the presence of an infant. (*Blue Jay's Dance* 44)

This difficulty of expression explains the scarcity of first person accounts. That Pauline's labor and delivery is given from the first person point of view is surely attributable in part to her personality. Her enormous mental will and her commitment to the mortification of her own flesh make her well-suited to remembering and relating the event. Pauline's Catholicism (she becomes the indomitable Sister Leopolda) leads her to treat labor as a form of penance or purification. The one paragraph we are given, however, could suffice for many labors:

Words were useless. Thoughts foolish. All of the mind's constructions. Time passed slowly because the pain was predictable, fast because it was a brimming well. I was slapped by a great beast, thrown over its shoulder, shaken like a child in the grip of its mother. I marveled at the breath torn out of me. I heard my own cries. Bernadette's voice bloomed and faded in my ear, telling me to do things, where to put my legs, when to suffer the humiliations of her touch. She instructed me to hold my breath or release, and finally, to push the child out with all my remaining strength. (134)

Several features of her comments are noteworthy, but especially her realization that words, thoughts, the mind's constructions are completely useless and foolish in these circumstances. The laboring mother is a slave to her body's will, utterly helpless. Erdrich sympathizes with this, writing "There are certain frustrations in approaching such an event, a drama in which the body stars and not the fiction-making mind. . . . I want to control the tale. I can't . . ." (*Blue Jay's Dance* 43). This may be one reason why we are taught to "suppress its importance over time, to devalue and belittle an experience in which we are bound up in the circular drama of human fate" (*Blue Jay's Dance* 44). Pauline is certainly mortified by her lack of bodily control. Tess Cosslett, too, in *Women Writing Childbirth,* expresses the near impossibility of representing the body's experiences: "It is only audience point of view narratives that are able to give single and simple accounts of childbirth: experienced from the centre, that 'centre' becomes diffuse, multiple, fractured" (118).

Erdrich does not rectify this situation in her fiction, which is to say she does not exalt the mother's body in the "circular drama of human fate" nor provide us with a "diffuse, multiple, fractured" narrative. What she does instead is to dramatize the various characters' reactions to the birth drama through "audience point of view narratives." Erdrich suggests that birth stories often become "paradigm and parable" (*Blue Jay's Dance* 44), thereby becoming the child's story rather than the mother's story. Erdrich's other fictional birth stories, those other than Pauline's that is, become paradigms or parables that tie the raw materials, the strands of the event, into a net that holds the individual safe. These paradigms are not just created for the child, but often for those who witness the birth. Characters' constructions of birth tales meet a set of narrative or rhetorical needs that consistently uphold a maternal ethos.

Erdrich's birth stories have a significant ability to connect an individual to other people in a web of family, community, or clan, functioning not so much as creation myths, but rather as connection myths. They explain the basis for connections between people, often people who on the surface have little in common. Erdrich seems loath to leave any of her characters disconnected; there is a compulsion in the novels toward bringing people home. Hertha Wong discusses this desire for connection in her essay "Adoptive Mothers and Thrown-Away Children in the Novels of Louise Erdrich." She cites Erdrich's interview with Bruchac in which she discusses the mixed-blood person's search for origins, for community, but Wong also attributes Erdrich's concentration on the "interconnectedness of all life" to her Chippewa heritage (Wong 191). As a mother, a mixed blood, and as a Chippewa, Erdrich possesses compelling reason for inquiring into the mysteries of birth, origin, and connection.

Birth is by definition an act of connection with another (even as, paradoxically, the mother and child disconnect). It is the basis for human relation. If any one thing could be said for Erdrich's novels it is that they exhibit an uncommon obsession with relationship at the literal and figurative levels. All five novels revolve around a set group of people with Fleur, Pauline, Dot, and Lipsha appearing most frequently. Genealogical charts of the characters are most easily drawn in web fashion or perhaps in a three-dimensional tree because the characters are so interrelated. Tracing birth in such an interrelated group of people takes on dual importance; it both reminds you of your place among all your relations and keeps you from marrying your half brother. Intermarriage was traditionally carefully monitored among tribal groups. Uusally indidividuals could neither marry within the same family nor the same clan. As those clan structures broke down, however, people had to keep track informally, not a simple task when women often bore children to more than one man. The birth story helps a small community or tribe keep track of its interrelationships and also provides one's place in the hierarchy of family groupings.

Another way in which Erdrich reveals her preoccupation with relationship is through coincidence. Coincidences abound in the novels, particularly in the climactic scene of *Tales of Burning Love* when Jack Mauser is led by his dead first wife June Morrissey back to the car which holds her son, Lipsha, who, in turn, is holding Jack's son, John. Meanwhile, down the road sit Jack's four other ex-wives with hitchhiker (and Dot's real husband) Gerry Nanapush stashed in the back of the red Explorer. Either Erdrich has a Dickens complex or she's writing about human interconnection, about a compulsion to bring people together, to relate them. The birth narratives in the novels actually help to ground characters in these relationships. They tell the story of how the characters belong. Without those stories, characters drift. Furthermore, when characters drift, the community falls apart. Children are left in the woods, left with adoptive mothers, or simply left to die. As adults, those children cannot make meaningful connections with others, nor take their rightful place in the family and community. Erdrich's fictive birth stories are literally about reconnecting, even recreating a disintegrating community. Erdrich wants to draw in her drifting characters, the June Morrisseys and Jack Mausers, to teach them their origins and bring them home.

The best example of this use of the birth narrative, and the type probably most people are familiar with, is Lulu's birth story. The segments of *Tracks* that are told from Nanapush's point of view are his attempts to reconcile Lulu to her mother Fleur and, by extension, to all her people. Lulu has just returned from boarding school and feels nothing but resentment for her mother and alienation from the community. Nanapush weaves a story that gives her a place in the web. "You were born on the day we shot the last bear, drunk, on the reservation" (58). Nanapush constructs the story around three days: the two Fleur is in labor, culminating with the bear's barging into the cabin and Lulu popping out, and the naming day when Father Damien arrives to baptize Lulu and record her birth in the Church records. The third day is significant to Nanapush in particular because he gives her his name. The story ties Lulu to her mother and her relatives in a number of ways. Discussing those present at the birth (Margaret, Pauline, Eli, Nanapush, Father Damien, and the bear) tells the child of her significance to them, of their care for her, their anxiety over her well-being. The child is further tied to her mother through knowledge of Fleur's great suffering in labor and delivery and the certainty that Fleur almost died in the process.

Lulu is tied to the larger cosmos of the reservation—all her relations—by knowing that she was born when the last bear died.

Even further, Nanapush connects Lulu to his own family in naming her: "I thought about my wives, especially White Beads and our daughter . . . I had kept a good blaze going for the women in the cabin by splitting wood until I thought the stringy muscles in my arms would burst. There were so many tales, so many possibilities, so many lies. The waters were so muddy I thought I'd give them another stir. 'Nanapush,' I said. 'And her name is Lulu'" (61). Thus Lulu carries on the Nanapush clan, one that would have otherwise died out. It is her trickster son, Gerry, who carries the Nanapush name forward. Lulu also bears the weight of all the deceased Pillagers on her shoulders. Fleur and Moses alone have survived the dying time (of rampant epidemic) and between them they have only Lulu (and later Gerry). In all, the story emphasizes Lulu's connection to the old clans and to traditional values, but it is also a story about hardship and survival. Fleur has sent Lulu away because she so feared for Lulu's life on the reservation. Significantly, Lulu not only survives; she becomes an abundant source of life, bearing sons by six different men and becoming a community leader as an elder.

Birth stories need not only be about the birth child's connection to the larger family though. In *The Beet Queen* Wallace Pfef tells the story of Dot Adare's birth, a story not of Dot's connection to the family but of Wallace's connection. A lonely, gay man in a North Dakota town, Wallace has no family nearby and his lover, Karl Adare, leaves him and takes up with Celestine. Nonetheless, the two are connected through Karl when a dog's barking forces him to look outside during a blizzard. There he finds Celestine in the throes of labor in a snowdrift outside his door. His story focuses largely on the careful preparations he makes: boiling water, sterilizing scissors, fetching sheets and towels, making a bed for the baby in a laundry basket. He tells of his own calm strength in the face of this astounding event occurring on his new sofa. The delivery is perfectly normal and the baby appears "ready," "formidable" (154). Celestine surprises him by insisting that the baby be named for him, finally after a day's thought settling on Wallacette. "As her male sponsor, I was glad to give her full name for the church records, and her date of birth. But when it came to the names of her parents I paused. I had to gather myself before I said them without a tremble" (155). Wallace takes on the role of father for the baby nicknamed Dot, doing everything from birthday parties to buying her the title of Beet Queen with the same competency he exhibits at her birth. Dot's birth also connects Wallace to Celestine of course, and, further, to Aunt Mary Adare. The three become co-parents to Dot. Wallace is alone no more, but a member of a family and even tied in a way to his old lover, the girl's biological father. Once again, we have the theme of connections in a web-like structure that transcends sexuality, gender, and generations.

Moving over time Erdrich presents us with a new generation in the process of regeneration but also with a rhetorical variation. The story of Dot Adare's pregnancy and childbirth is told by Albertine Johnson. Albertine's narrative purpose is less to tell about herself than it is to tell about Dot and Gerry. Albertine first meets Dot when Dot threatens her with a knife after seeing Albertine with Gerry. Later she ends up working the weigh shack (a truck-weighing station on the interstate highway) with Dot throughout Dot's pregnancy and beyond. Albertine's story helps to create/extend the myth of Gerry Nanapush since it is she who reports his partial escape act in impregnating Dot in the prison visiting room; breaking out of prison just as Dot is going into labor; and jumping from a third-story hospital window, squeezing through an impossibly small space and landing mostly unharmed on a police car after the baby is born. Albertine understands that it is the baby's birth that impels him to run, for "It was perhaps the very first time in his life he had something to run for" (168).

The story also tells, however, about Dot's anger over having to go through the pregnancy alone: "She knit his absences into thick little suits for the child, suits that would have stopped a truck on a dark road with their colors" (163). Even so, it is the baby that best expresses the couple: "She was so dense with life, such a powerful distillation of Dot and Gerry" (171). In this story, Albertine is recording a family, one to which she is deeply connected by kin ties to Gerry, and through physical and emotional proximity to Dot and Shawn. During Dot's labor, Gerry roars up on a motorcycle to pick Albertine up because Dot has asked for her. Albertine, the woman who has left the reservation for a college education, is still connected to this eccentric but powerful group of people. The proof is in Dot's request for her presence during labor. First perceived as a threat to the family, Albertine becomes a member of it.

We are provided with another family creation myth in Candice and Marlis's birth story in *Tales of Burning Love*. This story is one in which Candice initially treats the birth as a financial and legal arrangement with Marlis who alternately resists and gives in. As they spend time, "their unhappiness together seems warm, cozy, complete" (355). Candice experiences a sympathetic pregnancy and by the time Marlis goes into labor we find Candice threatening mayhem if the physician does not give Marlis pain relief. When Candice leads a sleep-deprived and crazed Marlis back to bed one night they end up making love. "Implications drifted over Candice and disappeared—she remembered vaguely that she had once regarded what seemed entirely normal, now, as absurd, foreign, freakish. The baby lay between the two of them" (360). They are a family. This story is told to the other two ex-wives in the midst of the blizzard, under the heading of tales of burning love intended to keep them all warm. The story's rhetorical purpose is essentially to announce their marriage. In this case family connection transcends not just gender and sexuality but also class and educational differences.

If those who have birth stories fare well, what happens to those who do not? The confirmation of this theory lies in the characters who lack a birth story or connection myth if you will—Jack, Karl Adare, and Lipsha Morrissey. All three men are cut off from their biological mothers in childhood. Jack's story is never fleshed out, but we are led to believe that he has been taken from his Indian mother who has periodic fits of depression and rage. Repressing his attachments to the land and his mother's people, Jack is only healed in the end of the novel when he accepts and nurtures his son on his mother's home reservation and accepts a job contract with Lyman Lamartine. Karl Adare is abandoned with Mary in the town of Argus when they are both children. While Mary situates herself adequately in her Aunt Fritzie's family, Karl hits the road and never looks back until middle age when he realizes he "wanted the whole world of people who belonged to each other" but after months of dissatisfaction, he realizes that what he "really wanted was their future. [He] wanted their children" (*The Beet Queen* 285). It is that desire for a future that leads Karl back to the messy complications of family. Finally, Marie Kashpaw never tells Lipsha who his mother is, when in actuality it is June Morrissey. While married to Gordie Kashpaw, June has had an affair with Gerry Nanapush, resulting in this pregnancy. Not wanting to disrupt the marriage, June asks Marie to raise the child outside its birth home. Lulu tells Lipsha the truth and reassures him that June had always "watched [him] from a distance" (*Love Medicine* 244). It is this knowledge that allows Lipsha to decide that he belongs to the family. "I was a real kid now, or halfway real" (255). Interestingly, it is most often the male characters who have difficulty with this sense of belonging.

Even the "thrown-away" girls in the novels still seek out family. Marlis has lost her mother as a child too and is raised by an abusive father, but she still recognizes her need for connection and family. June Morrissey's mother dies out in the bush, leaving June to wander, eating pine sap to survive. While her marriage to Gordie fails and she is hardly a model mother, she does make attempts to create family for herself. To some degree it is children—pregnancy, impending birth and babies—that necessitate the belonging to family for women. Raising children forces women to reach beyond themselves for help. In the world of Erdrich's novels, women are more likely to find that help from other women, not just in the midwives and birth attendants but also in lay healing and in the kind of assistance Marie offers by taking in children other women cannot raise.

While I have concentrated on how the birth narratives most often function as a means to tell or forge connections between people, the two stories which do not forge connection provide interesting case studies that help explain the centrality of these tales. The one story already mentioned is that of Pauline's delivery. Her story, the only one told from a mother's point of view, is about separation and loss. "If I gave birth, I would be lonelier" (*Tracks* 135). That one small sentence is the only hint we have of an alternative reading of the birth act for the birthing mother. In pregnancy the mother and child achieve the closest connection that two beings can have, such that there is often a blurring of identities. The rending of that connection is so profound that it often threatens both mother's and child's lives. The other story is that of Fleur's premature delivery which is also related by Pauline. Like Pauline, Fleur struggles to hold the baby inside her in order to save the "too soon" baby's life. After it slides from her, Fleur cuts the cord, breathes into the baby's mouth and wraps it tightly inside her shirt to her belly once more, almost as if she were trying to press it back inside.

In both of these stories, as in the postpartum depression that Marlis experiences, "her face savage and bewildered" (*Burning Love* 358), there are hints of the "conscious body" telling a birth story not about connection but about profound separation and loss, about mourning the loss of a perfect connection. For some mothers, and indeed for some entire cultures, the compulsion to reconnect may have its origins in that original separation. Cultures that honor a maternal sensibility—as Ojibwa culture does—may, in fact, be more predisposed to such an all-encompassing vision of one's relationship to the world.

Erdrich's birth story itself—a book-length narrative of pregnancy, delivery, and new motherhood—speaks to this complex relationship between the mind's desires and the body's imperatives.

First she was part of me, and then she slept curled between us. Then, a night, I don't know when, she was placed in her bassinet. Now she sleeps in the next room. For nights I wake, startled, my brain humming with abysmal exhaustion, aware only in the most atavistic way that something is wrong. It is as if in sleep I have been cut in two and suddenly I miss my other half. (*Blue Jay's Dance* 152)

It is at least in part that separation, that profound loss or its fear that drives many of Erdrich's plots. Like the mother stumbling down the dark hallway toward her crying newborn, her lost characters falter their way toward home, the place of belonging, where others know their stories, their origins. It is the mother's desire to meet that child's need that cries out for a community in which all are related, compelled by their birth to sustain the web, to keep others from falling away.

These birth stories actually approach a kind of sociological statement that is unusual for Erdrich. She is often noted for a quality to her writing that is sometimes called magical or symbolic realism, particularly within death scenes, (such as those of Henry Lamartine, Jr., and June Morrissey), or in natural disasters, (e.g., the windstorm that flattens Argus, North Dakota). In contrast, she treats childbirth, a key moment in the natural cycle and laden with symbolic overtones, in realistic terms. While not exaggerated or prolonged, the scenes offer pain, blood, despair, joy, and many of the other elements common to real-life births. Birth is not treated as metaphor for the creative process, nor as sacred ritual or transformative act, but rather as one of the hardest and most treacherous jobs a woman can ever perform. In *Blue Jay's Dance* she calls it "women's work" (42).

Erdrich takes birth *seriously,* refusing to place laurels on the heads of her women characters or flatter them as fertility goddesses. She shows how physically and emotionally taxing the process is and allows readers to draw their conclusions based on that. Erdrich's birth scenes are tied to realism in two respects. One, the shift in birthing practices is historically accurate over the course of the ninety years or so that are depicted in the novels. She moves from home births attended by lay midwives to hospital births and finally to birthing centers, reflecting the shifting trends of the twentieth century. Two is in the variety she brings to the birth scenes; no two scenes or circumstances leading to the birth are the same. Some characters labor for days, some for hours; some characters are intense, loving mothers and others more ambivalent; and some women have family to support and celebrate the baby's arrival, some have no one.

Judith Walzer Leavitt records the historical shift from early American practices of childbirth as assisted by female family, friends and the local midwife to, in the late nineteenth century and early twentieth century, depending upon the woman's financial status, physician-assisted births in the home and finally to hospital births which routinely excluded all "outside" support. Leavitt's sources indicate that immigrant and poor women in the United States frequently moved very late to hospital births and instead held onto female-assisted home births. Part of the reticence was financial, but a greater part of the women's reluctance was due to modesty. Similar constraints were reported by Ojibwa women to M. Inez Hilger in her research of the 1930s among Ojibwa people of Northern Minnesota, Wisconsin, and Michigan. "Midwives (*gat niwi kwe,* a term also used for any woman administering to the sick) usually attended the mother at birth. At times, however, only the woman's mother and sister, or some women who were near relatives, did" (12). One of Hilger's sources reported:

"I myself think it is a disgrace the way women submit themselves to strangers today when their babies are born, especially to those doctors. . . . In old days not even the women looked at anyone more than necessary; a big piece of buckskin was placed over the mother to protect her modesty." (12)

Such is the case with Fleur Pillager in *Tracks* when she gives birth to Lulu in the spring of 1914, laboring within the "birth house" with Margaret Kashpaw and Pauline attending her. Her husband Eli Kashpaw and Nanapush wait outside, not allowed in the house at all. Fleur labors for several days before a drunken bear barges through the cabin door: "[W]hen Fleur saw the bear in the house she was filled with such fear and power that she raised herself on the mound of blankets and gave birth" (*Tracks* 60). After the birth Margaret administers traditional remedies, packing wormwood and moss between Fleur's legs, wrapping her in stone-heated blankets, kneading her stomach and forcing down cups of boiled raspberry leaf tea.

Later in the same novel, around 1919, Pauline labors and delivers a baby within the home of the midwife/nurse with whom she lives and works, Bernadette Morrissey. Earlier in the pregnancy, Pauline has attempted some of the same kinds of methods to induce miscarriage that are reported by Hilger's informants, jumping from trees and hitting her belly. Pauline throws herself again and again on the handle of an axe until Bernadette stops her. Pauline has knowledge of an "old-time traditional," Moses Pillager, who could give her abortifacient "medicines of pounded roots and barks" (*Tracks* 132). A number of Hilger's sources spoke of an "Indian medicine which is made by steeping roots or herbs" that could abort a fetus (10). While Hilger's sources do not mention use of any kind of forceps-like device, Bernadette does use a device that looks to Pauline like two iron spoons that lock together in order to extract the baby from her. Leavitt's research found over a hundred variations of forceps in wide use by the latter half of the 1800s. Undoubtedly, the midwives adopted and modified many of these same practices/ devices over time.

Dot Adare's birth in *The Beet Queen* reveals a radically different notion of childbirth taking place in 1954. Dot's mother, Celestine, stays at home for much of her labor and then tries to drive herself to the hospital when the delivery draws near. After crashing into a snowbank and stumbling to a nearby house, she lies in the snow yelling until Wallace Pfef discovers her. Here is another home birth, although an unintentional one, with a male attending. After the delivery—a normal one with a good outcome for mother and child—they call the hospital nonetheless where Celestine and baby are taken the next morning. This reflects the thinking of the mid-twentieth century that saw childbirth as pathological, in need of medical intervention. It also reveals the lack of a knowledgeable cohort of women who could have supported Celestine in labor and delivery and would have been readily available a generation earlier.

In *Love Medicine* we have the capable Dot giving birth herself in a hospital in 1980. This scene is complete with the father pacing the waiting room and the close friend and shirttail relation, Albertine Johnson, also waiting outside. Here the medical community has completely taken over the birth scene and friend and family alike are excluded. Gerry is only invited in for a half-hour visit. Finally, in 1994, *Tales of Burning Love* starts to bring the birthing room scene back around to where women have some voice. Candice is allowed in the hospital room as Marlis's coach. When the doctor refuses to administer pain medication though because he likes "to follow the patient's instructions" Candice explodes, grabbing the doctor by the shirt and saying: "'You get the *epidural now or I'll kill you with my bare hands*'" (356, author's emphasis). It is not, however, until she hands him her attorney's card that he orders the epidural, showing women reasserting control in the birthing process, albeit ironically through the threat of litigation rather than through superior knowledge.

These scenes dramatize Leavitt's historical evidence that women's attempts to make childbirth safer and less painful actually backfired. Ironically, Leavitt argues, women abdicated their power over the birthing room, although other interpretations hold that physicians wrested the control away from women. During the nineteenth century women had near total authority over the doctors they invited to attend childbirth, yet in the late twentieth century doctors have taken control. Women have to act aggressively to reassert any authority. The scenes also reflect trends away from traditional customs, herbal medicines, and family-centered births. Much more often than not, women "submit themselves to strangers" (Hilger 12) in places far from home.

Even within this historically determined context, the birth scenes exhibit tremendous variety, just as real births do. In *Blue Jay's Dance*

Erdrich comments that "Every birth is profoundly original" (46). We could expect nothing less than original birth scenes from such a profoundly original writer. Fleur Pillager's first pregnancy is the result of gang rape, the biological father undetermined. Her second pregnancy, though conceived with her spouse Eli Kashpaw, ends in premature delivery and the baby's death. Fleur nearly dies as well. Pauline gets pregnant as a result of satisfying her sexual curiosity with Napoleon Morrissey. Celestine's pregnancy results from a short-lived romantic liaison with Karl Adare. Dot and Gerry make love just out of view of the closed circuit TV in the prison visiting room, thereby creating Shawn. Marlis's pregnancy is also within the bonds of matrimony but utterly unwanted by the father, Jack Mauser. Babies are conceived in and out of matrimony, in violence, in lust, in love.

Some of the babies are wanted: Fleur dotes on Lulu, although a product of rape, and Fleur struggles prodigiously to save her prematurely born infant. She even goes to the land of the dead to gamble for the lives of her children. Some infants are despised: Pauline tries to hold the baby within so that the two of them will die together. Seeing the child after Bernadette wrenches it out of her, Pauline thinks she is "soiled, formed by me, bearing every defilement I had known by Napoleon Morrissey" (*Tracks* 136). Some mothers are deeply ambivalent: Marlis, after bearing John, Jr., in *Tales of Burning Love,* cries for weeks because she cannot decide whether or not to give the child up for adoption. June Morrissey is ambivalent—although she gives up the baby Lipsha for another woman to raise (in *Love Medicine*), after her own death she saves Lipsha by guiding Jack Mauser to the car where Lipsha and John, Jr., are stranded in the blizzard (in *Burning Love*). The women who are most settled in their identity and their connections to family seem to be the most secure about pregnancy and the coming of children—Fleur, Dot, Celestine. In Marlis's case she has no family, an unsupportive husband, and no steady source of income so she would be foolish if she were not worried about the pregnancy.

Pauline's case would seem to indicate that the unconditional love of babies is tied on some level in Erdrich's mind to a rejection of Catholicism. Pauline has two reasons for wanting the child to die within her. One is selfish—she can see no future for herself except a lonely one once the child is born: "I would be an outcast, a thing set aside for God's use, a human who could be touched by no other human" (*Tracks* 135). The other reason entails original sin, a hatred for her own sexuality and for the body in general. Pauline, of course, has a future as Sister Leopolda, nun with a vengeance, so her thinking is often tortured and extreme. It is, however, significant that the character who defends her children to the death also defends Pillager land, lives in the old ways, and speaks to the old Ojibwa spirits. The character who would deny her own children their birth, suffocating them in her womb, is a Catholic convert and Fleur's nemesis.

In two stories Erdrich indicates a sense that pregnancy is a time of great power for women, despite their physical vulnerability. Two characters who experience pregnancy as a time of despair—Pauline and Marlis—go to great lengths to exercise their power over others. Pauline manipulates Eli and Sophie into having sex as a way of exorcizing her jealousy of Fleur and her rejection by Eli. Marlis is herself rejected by Jack when she tells him she is pregnant. In an effort to force Jack's attention and exact a little revenge, Marlis duct tapes him to a hotel bed and proceeds to show him the pain she goes through for him: plucking his eyebrows, hot waxing his legs, applying spike heels to his feet with super glue, putting brush curlers in his hair. When Jack refuses to tell Marlis he loves her and is happy about the baby, she puts duct tape over his mouth and leaves him for some hotel maid to find. These may be hormonal surges, but in both cases the women are acting desperately out of their isolation at a time when they very much need love and reassurance.

Erdrich is so careful about providing every conceivable type of birth situation that we even get birth stories from several characters who cannot physically give birth. Nanapush relates:

Many times in my life, as my children were born, I wondered what it was like to be a woman, able to invent a human from the extra materials of her own body. In the terrible times, the evils I do not speak of, when the earth swallowed back all it had given me to love, I gave birth in loss. I was like a woman in my suffering, but my children were all delivered into death. It was contrary, backward, but now I had a chance to put things into a proper order. (*Tracks* 167)

Nanapush stays awake all night singing and warming the half-frozen Lulu Nanapush, his namesake child, delivering her from death and back into life. A trickster like Nanapush, Lipsha too can embrace the feminine. When caught in the blizzard with John, Jr., in *Tales of Burning Love,* Lipsha slips the baby inside his shirt against his belly to keep him warm. When Jack saves Lipsha from the car he does not realize he has also saved his son until he hears a wail and Lipsha gives birth, unzipping his jacket to reveal the baby "tiny, raw, screaming, red" (387), for all the world like a newborn. In Erdrich's most recent novel, *The Antelope Wife,* Scranton Roy breast feeds both the Ojibwa baby he has rescued and his own son. His observations upon the birth of his son reveal him to be deeply sympathetic to women and their efforts to create and sustain life: "Scranton wrapped the baby in the skin of a dog and kissed the smoothed, ravaged temples of Peace with tender horror at the pains of his own mother, and of all mothers, and of the unfair limitations of our bodies, of the hopeless settlement of our life tasks, and finally, of the boundless iniquity of the God to whom she had so uselessly shrieked" (17). The most admirable men in Erdrich's novels know how to effect those loving and life-giving connections with children, with other people. Characters like Jack need to learn.

These birth narratives remain grounded in realism for several reasons. One is that, as I have argued, the characters need grounding in a story that firmly and realistically connects them to others, to family, to community. The stories are too important to leave their interpretation to chance and therefore they call upon verifiable historical detail. Even Nanapush, who is willing to further muddy the waters by giving Lulu his name, is careful to tell Lulu the real facts of her origins as far as he knows them.

Two, Erdrich flatly refutes any primitivist fantasy of Indian women's childbirth. Fleur is by far the most traditional and perhaps the strongest Ojibwa woman in the novels. She survives the epidemic that kills off most of her family and the surrounding community. She lives in the woods on her own, is said to communicate with the old gods, supposedly raises the windstorm that flattens Argus, and arranges to have the forest fall down upon the loggers who come to seize her home. Still, this paragon of supernatural strength requires two days of agonizing labor, in a house, on a bed, with two attendants, and finally the threat of a bear bursting into the room before she delivers her child. There is no question of her squatting behind a tree and resuming work. Fleur's niece, Celestine, also described as very large and capable, would freeze in a snowbank without the help of Wallace Pfeff. In fact, none of the deliveries described in the novels, including Nanapush's and Lipsha's, are easy. They all entail prolonged suffering and fear of death.

Three, these birth stories may also reflect historical realities because Erdrich herself is in some ways tied to the discourses of those birthing patterns. In *Women Writing Childbirth* Cosslett examines the degree to which women writers must still challenge the dominant discourses of childbirth, their voices "culturally constructed by prevailing discourses and cultural practices" (3). Erdrich's comments in *Blue Jay's Dance* reveal her careful consideration of a variety of birthing methods, from natural childbirth to conventional medical practices. Cosslett argues that women writers' attempts to negotiate those "prevailing ideologies" are tied to power: "in terms of writing, the power to take over the story, in terms of childbirth, the power to control the experience; or, in both cases, the power to protest, or celebrate, lack of control" (3). Erdrich's treatment of the birth scenes in her novels, then, may indicate her and her characters' power (or lack of power) over the experience, a power influenced by the historically shifting approaches to birth. Within the novels, as the birth process becomes further removed from the family and community, the story becomes increasingly distant until the mother almost disappears. With the appearance of Candice in the birthing room, there may be some reversal of this trend, but her story seems to emphasize a struggle between the medical community and the consumer, an institutionalized bedtime story for an alienated culture.[2]

The realism of the stories only underscores the fact that no matter how it happens, why it happens, where it happens or with whom, the essential separation of birth will compel us to reconnect with others in some meaningful way. Those with strong mother bonds have the advantage over those who lack them. Mothers, however, need the help of other women and of nurturant men in order to raise children with their identity and relationship to the world intact. Birth stories need not be created by the mother alone. Indeed, mothers may have limited verbal control over the event and so it may fall to witnesses to tell children of their origins. The mother's story of separation and loss is usurped by the child's story of entrance into the larger family and community, but understanding the mother's point of view helps to explain that longing for a perfect union that could only be sustained at the expense of life.

These novels represent a major literary contribution to that "intellectual quilt." Erdrich has been quietly pioneering birth stories, not just in the way that women experience and articulate their own labors and deliveries but in the broader social significance of the birth narrative as a source of regeneration and renewal of family, community, and clan. She joins an international group of women writers who are calling for a revaluation of maternal subjectivity. Our children and our future rest upon the outcome.

Notes

1. They inhabit Turtle Mountain Reservation area in North Dakota and are of mixed Ojibwa and European American descent. The novels span the last ninety years and, though the story is not told in chronological order, I have organized my discussion of them in chronological order within the novels rather than the order in which they were published to clarify the shifting cultural and historical conditions of childbirth. Erdrich's most recent novel, at the moment of

writing this essay, *The Antelope Wife,* focuses on an apparently unrelated multi-generational family of Ojibwa, German American, and Plains tribal people.

2. An interesting irony, perhaps unintentional, exists in this scene. Although Candice is present in the birthing room only because women have reasserted some control over it, Candice asks for the very thing—pain relief—that Leavitt argues led to the original loss of control over the birth process.

Works Cited

Cosslett, Tess. *Women Writing Childbirth: Modern Discourses of Motherhood.* Manchester, England: Manchester UP, 1994.

Erdrich, Louise. *The Beet Queen.* New York: Bantam, 1987.

——. "Birth." *Baptism of Desire.* New York: Harper Perennial, 1989. 63.

——. *The Blue Jay's Dance: A Birth Year.* New York: HarperCollins, 1995.

——. *Love Medicine.* New York: Bantam, 1984.

——. *Tales of Burning Love.* New York: HarperCollins, 1996.

——. *Tracks.* New York: Harper and Row, 1988.

Hilger, M. Inez. *Chippewa Child Life and Its Cultural Background.* St. Paul: Minnesota Historical Society Press, 1992. Reprinted from Smithsonian Institution Bureau of American Ethnology, 1951.

Leavitt, Judith Walzer. *Brought to Bed: Child-Bearing in America 1750-1950.* New York: Oxford UP, 1986.

Wong, Hertha D. "Adoptive Mothers and Thrown-Away Children in the Novels of Louise Erdrich." *Narrating Mothers:Theorizing Maternal Subjectivities.* Ed. Brenda O. Daly and Maureen T. Reddy. Knoxville: U of Tennessee P, 1991. 174-92.

9

"SOME EPIC USE FOR MY EXCELLENT BODY":

REDEFINING CHILDBIRTH AS HEROIC

IN *BELOVED* AND "THE LANGUAGE OF THE BRAG"

Ellen Argyros

With the wave of feminist scholars like Tess Cosslett, Marianne Hirsch, Margaret Homans and others who are exploring the issues of maternal subjectivity, the social construction of mothering, and the relationships between representation and reproduction, and with anthologies like Laura Chester's *Cradle and All: Women Writers on Pregnancy and Birth,* the birthing body is beginning to emerge as a legitimate subject of representation within the canon of American literature and theory. Indeed, Chester's book suggests that whole canons or bodies of literature are being formulated around the image of the body straining to expel another body. In Toni Morrison's novel *Beloved* and Sharon Olds' poem "The Language of the Brag," childbirth is not just represented in all its messy, bloody, corporeal reality; it is represented as a heroic achievement, no less worthy of praise than Achilles' slaying of Hector. These writers challenge us to examine our criteria regarding what constitutes a heroic act and reflect upon how and why birthing women have traditionally been excluded from the category of heroes. I have chosen to discuss these writers in particular precisely because they are so different: Olds is a European American poet who writes what might be called prosy poems, while Morrison is an African American novelist whose fiction is highly figural and poetic. Moreover, the literary forefathers to whom they address themselves present different models of authority, thereby provoking very different tonal responses from their literary daughters. Thus, the differences between Olds and Morrison suggest that a writer's interest in heroizing childbirth narratives transcends both her race and the genre in which she chooses to write.

As contemporary writers, Morrison and Olds are the beneficiaries of the modernist deconstruction of the notion of the hero as a larger than life male warrior who manages to transcend his physical limitations in order to destroy the bodies of his enemies and secure his own symbolic immortality through the fame accorded him by the poet, a fame which constitutes another kind of transcending of his body.[1]

Writers like Morrison and Olds, then, are engaged in the act of according new status to the body—and specifically to the birthing female body—and doing so in such a way as to suggest that this kind of transvaluation is needed if genocidal programs (like war, like slavery) are to be avoided. Olds and Morrison represent childbirth as heroic not only in order to valorize the experience of ordinary women, however. They do so in part to help insinuate themselves into a new and more inclusive American canon made up of male writers like Whitman and Ginsberg, and Faulkner and Twain. Olds' poem may further be read as a kind of playful critique of the Bloomian model of authorial anxiety. I would suggest that it is with one eye on their literary forefathers—toward whom they feel ambivalent, both indebted and defiant—that Olds and Morrison reevaluate the heroic and attempt to insinuate their texts into the larger American canon of literature.

How one defines heroic is critical here. The *New Shorter Oxford English Dictionary* defines hero as "a man, now also a woman, distinguished by the performance of extraordinarily brave or noble deeds [and] a man, now also a woman, admired and venerated for his or her achievements and noble qualities in a field." What I wish to draw attention to is that there are two components to the hero, according to this definition: there is the performance of a self-sacrificing, noble, honorable deed and then there is the public recognition which retrospectively identifies and reifies the act as having been heroic. The subjective element comes into play with those who interpret the act as heroic and with how much emphasis one places on the adverb "extraordinarily." Soldiers, traditionally male, risk death in great numbers to defend their personal honor and that of their country, but an individual woman quietly faces the possibility of death (for herself or for her child) every time she has a baby. If one defines a hero as someone who endures pain and risks death for some higher purpose, then a woman bearing a child might surely be classified as heroic, insofar as she risks her own life in order to initiate into existence a new member of the community. Childbearing is not just a personal act but a social one too. And while it is true that one might argue that there is nothing extraordinary about the sacrifices entailed in giving birth, given that childbirth is a "natural act" requiring endurance more than strategizing, I would claim that any time one knowingly risks one's life for some higher purpose that person is behaving extraordinarily.

In terms of the risks faced by pregnant women, Stephanie Shaw points out that infant mortality and infanticide were especially high for children of slaves in the antebellum south, remarking dryly that "the overall conditions of slavery were often not conducive to preserving the lives of slave children. While infant mortality rates generally declined over the decades, some mothers experienced death rates among their children that were as high just before the demise of slavery as they were at the end of the eighteenth century" (246). More generally, Judith Leavitt, in *Brought to Bed: Child-bearing in America 1750-1950,* estimates that in the early twentieth century one mother died for each 154 living births and that "deaths from maternity-related causes at the turn of the twentieth century were approximately 65 times greater than they were in the 1980s" (23-25). Leavitt describes the various fears that all women must have felt while undergoing childbirth:

Maternity, the creation of new life, carried with it the ever-present possibility of death. The shadow that followed women through their childbearing years was the fear of the physical risks of bearing children. Young women perceived that their bodies, even when healthy and vigorous, could yield up a dead infant or could carry the seeds of their own destruction. As Cotton Mather had warned at the beginning of the eighteenth century, and as many American women continued to believe, conception meant "your Death has Entered into you." Nine months of gestation could mean nine months to prepare for death. A possible death sentence came with every pregnancy. (20)

In addition to fearing that they might die in childbirth (whether of puerperal fever or some other cause), women had cause to fear that they would suffer agonizing and unremitting pain,[2] that their infants would die either in birth or within the years immediately following, that their bodies would be maimed for life (due to unsutured perineal tears, prolapsed uteri, or other causes), or that their recovery periods after childbirth would be unduly protracted, thus forcing post-parturient women to obtain extra household help (Leavitt 13-35). One woman, regarding her third birth in 1885, wrote: "Between oceans of pain there stretched continents of fear; fear of death and dread of suffering beyond bearing" (qtd. in Leavitt 33). Another wrote in 1877 that her third confinement brought "the nethermost hell of bodily pain and mental blankness" (qtd. in Leavitt 33). As late as 1934, a Dr. Joseph DeLee wrote of "the immense army of women suffering, if I may coin a phrase, subinvalidism and who say they have never felt well since their first baby was born" (qtd. in Leavitt 70).

It is perhaps not coincidental that Dr. DeLee invokes a military metaphor to describe the vast numbers of women who continue to suffer even after their children are born. Heroism, as I have noted, implies that an individual has managed to transcend the temptation to preserve his or her own personal comfort by risking pain and death for some larger cause. Similarly, the writer's act of describing a death-defying act (such as participating in a war or giving birth) helps to solidify the individual's achievement by insuring that the narrative of heroic achievement will live on after that body's demise.

Olds is keenly aware of the Homeric poet's social and cultural function in a time of war: to extol the reputation and insure the symbolic immortality of the mortal hero even while representing the physical immortality of the gods in the Olympian pantheon. If Olds wants to insure simultaneously both the honor of the birthing female and the power that she as poet has to assure that honor, Morrison is less gleefully defiant in her project: less combative, more quietly assertive. If Olds generally invokes a series of concentric circles (Homer and the Trojan War, Whitman and the Civil War, and a Bloomian War within the American Academy) as the historical contexts for her poem and for her sense of the heroic, Morrison keeps an unswerving eye on the specific conditions of life in the antebellum south and on slavery as an instrument of white patriarchal oppression for men and women—but especially for women. Perhaps in part since the poem is an older form than the novel (with a longer tradition of involvement with the identification of heroes and the preservation of their honor), and perhaps in part due to the temperaments of the two writers, Olds is more vehement, more adamant, and more explicit in her pronouncements about birthing as heroic while Morrison more quietly but powerfully dramatizes the heroism of Sethe.

Another important reason for the two writers' tonal differences has to do, of course, with their own complicated and ambivalent relationships to their "adversarial" literary forefathers. Olds is clearly annoyed at Whitman's and Ginsberg's assumptions that metaphors for procreation can somehow enable them as poets to transcend the limitations of their non-bearing bodies, while Morrison seems to feel some gratitude towards Twain and Faulkner for foregrounding the issue of race at all, even if they do so in a way that requires her patient revisions. Olds does active, sweaty battle with her literary forefathers; Morrison more matter-of-factly, more calmly goes about the business of subverting their assumptions because she is mindful of their courage in addressing race at all.

In "The Language of the Brag," Sharon Olds is far more overt and audacious than Morrison in both heroically representing childbirth and challenging her literary forefathers, Whitman and Ginsberg. Describing her own heroics of childbirth enables her to simultaneously establish a camaraderie with other American poets interested in celebrating the body and foreground the issue of gender difference as she mimics a tone of masculine bravado about how she can give birth while they cannot. "I have wanted some epic use for my excellent body,/some heroism, some American achievement," her persona announces and in the next breath confesses wistfully that "I have stood by the sandlot/and watched the boys play." By the end of the poem, the persona proclaims: "I have done what you wanted to do, Walt Whitman,/Allen Ginsberg . . . and I am putting my proud American boast/right here with the others." Clearly, the desire to be physically and emotionally tested is aligned with the desire for inclusion within the canon of male American poets who have foregrounded the male body in their works. With self-conscious bravado and in-your-face oneupmanship, Olds uses her own ability to bear children as a way of differentiating herself from Whitman and Ginsberg and implying that she is like them—only better—because she can generate both children and poems, both physical and symbolic immortality. Childbirth becomes rewritten as a privileged, heroic rite of passage that women engage in voluntarily, even defiantly.

It is worth noting that if Olds' one-upped literary forefathers were either admittedly gay or were thought to have harbored homoerotic desires, Morrison's were white males who have written extensively on race. Both Twain and Faulkner have the reputations of being comparatively pioneering white writers who addressed the knotty question of race relations, and Morrison eventually wrote her master's thesis on alienated figures in Woolf and Faulkner. There are, in addition, a number of pieces of internal evidence suggesting Faulkner's influence on Morrison's writing, to say nothing of the recent and compelling study by Philip Weinstein, *What Else But Love? The Ordeal of Race in Faulkner and Morrison*.[3] And, as has been noted, in *Playing in the Dark* she implies that she would have had good reason to want to rewrite the relationship between Huck and Jim. Whereas for Olds the challenge is to defy those poetic forefathers who can bear only symbolic children (and who therefore have an under-appreciation of the heroism required for the act of birth), for Morrison the challenge is to try to do what Twain could not: create a relationship between a white person and a black person that avoids objectifying or idealizing either one.

Whitman's and Ginsberg's roles as gay male American poets who celebrate the body is relevant on three accounts: it marks them as even less likely to inseminate a woman and thereby father a child than the average heterosexual male; it suggests that they might regard the act of love as an end in itself rather than a means to the end of procreation, and it suggests that the gendered body they fantasize about in their poetry is probably male. Olds, whose experience as a mother is an important subject of her poetry, seems both affronted and inspired by these features of their poetry and themselves.

The body in general has always been central to Olds' work. Although her most recent book of poetry focuses almost obsessively on the dying body of her father, Olds begins her poetic career preoccupied with the birthing body of the mother. In her earliest book of poems, *Satan Says* (1980), Olds includes a whole section of poems entitled "Mother," including "Young Mothers" I, II, IV, and V, and "The Language of the Brag." In *The Living and the Dead* (1983), she includes sections on The Family, The Men, and The Children—but none on the mother. Though categorically absent, the mother is, however, frequently present as the narrating persona of the poem, particularly in the section on children and also in the touching poem "New Mother," which depicts the relations between new parents after the birth of their first child. Her collection *The Gold Cell* takes its title from a poem within it entitled "The Quest," which details a mother's paranoid fears that linger after her daughter has been lost for an hour, and the book includes other poems from the perspective of the mother. In her most recent book of poetry, *The Father* (1992), Olds strays the farthest she ever has from the birthing body of the mother, for this latest collection of poetry is primarily a series of elegies for her late father. There are no sub-categories of poems; they are almost all devoted to describing the nuances of her feelings and revelations about this man's slow death to cancer. There are only a few rare allusions to the role of the procreative powers of the mother in this book of death. In "Nullipara" is the book's only reference to the anticipated birth of a child, and that child is, significantly, a stillborn.

In focusing on "The Language of the Brag," then, I return to an earlier Olds. The poem begins with the persona's expressing her desire for excellence in some physical accomplishment like the knife-throw; she desires this excellence not out of a feeling of lack, not because she is physically weak but because she feels herself to be exceptionally strong, and she wants public recognition for her strength: she wants "to achieve something at the center of a crowd." "I have wanted some epic use for my excellent body" initially suggests an allusion to the Greeks—to Homer's *Iliad,* for example—but then she identifies the desire for "some heroism, some American achievement" as if to specify an alliance between her desire and that of her relatively recently born country. Her voice changes from one of mock-bombast and chest-thumping to a quieter, more plaintive tone when she notes: "I have stood by the sandlot/ and watched the boys play." Suddenly, all the hyperbole drops away, and we are left with the image of a young girl's feelings of exclusion. By the next stanza, this persona has inflated herself again with the former tone, but this time she begins to enumerate what she has already done as a pregnant woman:

> ... I have dragged around
> my belly big with cowardice and safety,
> my stool black with iron pills,
> my huge breasts oozing mucus ...
> I have lain down and sweated and shaken
> and passed blood and feces and water and
> slowly alone in the center of a circle I have
> passed the new person out ...
> I have done what you wanted to do, Walt Whitman,
> Allen Ginsberg, I have done this thing,
> I and the other women this exceptional
> act with the exceptional human body,
> this giving birth, this glistening verb,
> and I am putting my proud American boast
> right here with the others. (Olds 44-45)

After the initial expressions of longing, the persona realizes that, ironically, she and other women have already done something monumental, courageous, worth singing about. Olds argues that both pregnancy and childbirth be viewed as heroic, for they require that the individual endure great suffering, that she adapt herself to the grotesque transformation of her body as the first of many self-sacrifices, and that she risk her life as she lies "alone on a bed,/sweating, isolated by pain,/splitting slowly." Olds' redefinition of the heroic daringly privileges the life-affirming act of childbirth over the more destructive damage to the body sustained in war.

In another poem from *Satan Says,* "Nurse Whitman," Olds draws our attention to Whitman's nurturing relationship to the wounded bodies of soldiers during the Civil War, as she imagines herself working alongside him and repairing the bodies:

> ... the male bodies in beds.
> We bend over them, Walt, taking their breath
> soft on our faces, wiping their domed brows, stroking back the
> coal-black Union hair.
> We lean down, our pointed breasts
> heavy as plummets with fresh spermy milk—
> we conceive, Walt, with the men we love, thus, now,
> we bring to fruit. (13)

First Olds' speaker identifies Whitman in his traditionally feminine role of nurse, which he occupied during the Civil War, tenderly caring for soldiers, writing letters for them, notifying their parents of their deaths. She situates herself alongside him and addresses him familiarly as they minister to soldiers' bodies. Then her body and Whitman's body become the foci of attention as she begins to impose upon his the image of "pointed breasts" full of "fresh spermy milk." Gender becomes confused, conflated, immaterial: both nurses are full of nourishing, creative liquid—the spermy milk evokes the associated image of sperm whales, Moby Dick, and the exclusive canon of male American literature not far away from this poem—which will be used to both nourish the men and conceive poetry inspired by the men, conception being a pun on both the ability to comprehend (the pain of others) and the ability to create and procreate with others something new. Olds identifies with the idealistic Whitman, who both valorized camaraderie and nursed the wounded casualties of those dying boys at the front, but then triumphantly declares that she can both celebrate the body and give life to new ones. Her boasting in a rather shameless fashion about her unique prowess as an Amazonian birther only enhances her mock-bravado, showing that she can subvert through mimicry those who privilege death-dealing bodies over life-giving ones.

Olds' emphasis is on the relationship between the woman and her body, and the newfound confidence she has in it and in herself after she has given birth. The excretions of the body are viewed as signs of her ennobling pain, and death is present not as a real threat but only as a means of helping to valorize the act. Childbirth becomes transfigured from a natural act to an act requiring Homeric courage. Olds uses all this chest-thumping about the trials of pregnancy and childbirth as a way to jockey for power within a male tradition and as a way to taunt the likes of Whitman and Ginsberg for their comparative lack of fecundity. But if Olds' birthing mother seems to do so by a kind of willed parthenogenesis—for her partner is never mentioned and she does not admit to feeling dependent on anyone else throughout the process—Morrison's Sethe is in an extraordinarily vulnerable situation. Her husband's having mysteriously disappeared, Sethe is on the brink of giving birth unattended by the side of a river when she is discovered by the passing Amy Denver.

In *Beloved,* Morrison pays quiet tribute to the heroism of the fugitive slave, Sethe, who gives birth in the woods. One could not imagine a less desirable context in which to give birth. Sethe is physically and emotionally exhausted with the ordeal of "trying to get to her three children, one of whom was starving for the food she carried" (31). Her husband has disappeared; she has suffered a kind of lactation rape at the hands of two white boys, and now she sees what appears to be another white boy. Amy Denver is "the raggediest-looking trash you ever saw" (32) and is hungry. Initially, she is on an immediate quest for huckleberries; then she speaks of a larger quest for carmine velvet. To Amy's meandering train of thought which culminates in a question—"Thought there'd be huckleberries. Look like it. That's why I come up in here. Didn't expect to find no nigger woman. If they was any, birds ate em. You like huckleberries?"—Sethe replies "I'm having a baby, miss." Amy reluctantly accepts the position of unofficial midwife, even though it is pathetically clear that she has no qualification for the position, having never given birth herself nor assisted anyone else, although she is "good at sick things" (82).

The huckleberry exchange, an easily overlooked detail of the novel, is worth some attention. Amy's hunger makes her so obsessed with finding something to eat that she seems initially oblivious to Sethe's condition. Sethe reminds her—gently, deferentially—that she is about to give birth, implying that this state of affairs necessitates new priorities for both of them, if Amy chooses to help her. Amy is still rather obtuse to Sethe's need when she remarks "That mean you don't have no appetite? Well I got to eat me something" (32). She still does not get it. She then begins discussing her quest for carmine velvet in Boston. What is striking here is the association Morrison makes between the kind of elusive fruit Amy is seeking and the character Huckleberry Finn. Both Amy and Huck Finn are described by their respective authors as "white trash"; both are hungry and scrawny; both are invested in their antithetically symmetrical quests (for velvet/bourgeois respectability, for a kind of freedom which is defined in negation to bourgeois respectability); both speak a similar dialect and are blunt to the point of rudeness at times; both have been physically beaten by persons in authority over them; both wander about in the wilderness; yet both also possess a kind of scrappy survival instinct. Morrison introduces the huckleberry at a point in the narrative where Amy has to be reminded that Sethe is in an even more vulnerable situation than herself, that Sethe is about to give birth and, therefore, needs attention. From a moral standpoint, Amy cannot simply pretend she is a kind of female Huck with no responsibilities to anyone else now; with some reluctance, Amy is forced to recognize that what she needs to do is to minister to Sethe because their similarities transcend their differences. Finally, Sethe's condition draws Amy out of herself and the two "throw-away people" do their work "appropriately and well" (85).

If one reads *Beloved* alongside Morrison's critical study *Playing in the Dark: Whiteness and the Literary Imagination,* published five years afterward, one can see that in her fiction Morrison rewrites Twain's representation of the interracial river-side friendship between Huck and Jim in her description of the relationship between Sethe and her unlikely midwife-attendant Amy Denver. In her critical work, Morrison suggests why she might have done so: so as to underscore some of the limitations of Twain's narrative—especially its objectifying of Jim as an "invisible other" with an "apparently limitless store of love and compassion . . . for his white friend" even when Huck proves unspeakably cruel (56). Commenting specifically on the ending of *Huckleberry Finn,* Morrison writes that:

The humiliation that Huck and Tom subject Jim to is baroque, endless, foolish, mind-softening—and it comes after we have experienced Jim as an adult, a caring father and a sensitive man. If Jim had been a white ex-convict befriended by Huck, the ending could not have been imagined or written: because it would not have been possible for two children to play so painfully with the life of a white man (regardless of his class, education, or fugitiveness) once he had been revealed to us as a moral adult. (*Playing* 54-57)

Jim's manipulation by the text into a selfless moral guide for Huck is objectionable on aesthetic as well as moral grounds, for it results in Twain's falsifying through idealization the relationship between black man and white boy. Part of Morrison's agenda seems to be to suggest that of the two sets of outlaws—Twain's and hers—the women accomplish a feat that is similar to but more heroic than what the men do. Sethe and Amy use the river not so much to escape from the authorities and, therefore, save themselves so much as they risk being caught in order to save the infant's life. Sethe knows that she could just give herself up to exhaustion and die, but she does not have the luxury of doing so; to do so would be to relegate her child to being buried alive. In *Beloved,* Morrison is situating herself explicitly next to her white literary forefathers like Twain and Faulkner, but doing so in such a way as to underscore the limitations of their narratives in expressing black female experience.

Morrison, in her assessment of *Huckleberry Finn,* enters into an already existing debate about the extent to which this novel may be viewed as a serious critique of slavery and racism, a fundamentally racist text, or some hybrid of the two. Without entering too deeply into this complex debate, I would simply like to draw attention to the perspective and prose style of one other African American scholar writing about the treatment of race in Twain's novel. Julius Lester, in his essay "Morality and *Adventures of Huckleberry Finn,*" critiques this novel as representing a white American adolescent male fantasy "that freedom from

restraint and responsibility represents paradise" (qtd. in Graff 347).⁴
Lester also notes that civilization in Twain's novel "is equated with education, regularity, decency and being 'cramped up,' and the representa-
tives of civilization are women" (qtd. in Graff 346). More interestingly,
throughout his essay Lester draws upon figurative language which cor-
porealizes the mother's body that is so conspicuously missing in Twain's
novel: Lester begins by noting that "Tom and Huck are part of our American selves, a mythologem we imbibe with our mother's milk" (qtd. in
Graff 341); he goes on to note that "too many other white American
males . . . persist in clinging to the teat of adolescence long after only
blood oozes from the nipples. They persist in believing that freedom
from restraint and responsibility represents paradise" (qtd. in Graff 347).

Lester's critique is relevant to my argument because he foregrounds
how Twain's novel valorizes "freedom from restraint and responsibility,"
because he observes that the feminine is equated with the numbing constraints of civilization, and because he suggests through his metaphors
that the body of the mother—her milk, her breasts, her nipples—is dangerously absent in Twain's novel. Morrison's achievement in lovingly
reconstituting the parts of that body, acknowledging that women are
more captive to their bodies than men are, and re-valorizing the importance of responsibility (which is what no mother can escape from either
before, during, or after the birth of her child) is all the more impressive
when seen in the light of Lester's reading of *Huckleberry Finn* as a
hymn to male adolescent values. If *Huckleberry Finn* is a hymn to male
adolescent values, *Beloved* is clearly a hymn to female post-parturient
ones.

Chance, luck, and his own sheer cleverness help Huck survive in a
threatening world of abusive fathers, opportunistic tramps, and meddling
older women who force one into starchy clothes. Sethe endures her
ordeals with some luck, with some intuition of who can be trusted, and
significantly without the strong faith in God that her mother-in-law Baby
Suggs possesses before she becomes disillusioned. We may not expect a
young boy like Huck to be sustained by spiritual faith, but—with the
example of Faulkner's Dilsey in mind—we might expect a female slave
to cling to some hope of divine protection in an otherwise pitiless world.
Yet Sethe conspicuously does not pray.

There may be a God in Morrison's novel, but Sethe does not make
any appeals to him. Morrison's representation of Sethe's giving birth
with the help of Amy Denver is triangulated by the mediating presence
of God, first with the semi-facetious line "Amy stopped begging Jesus
and began to curse His daddy" and then with the more serious line "the
wet sticky women clambered ashore to see what, indeed, God had in

mind" (84). When the fate of Sethe and her children is not being determined directly by the white slave owners, it is being determined by the divine patriarchal authority whose intents are not always clear. If there are no threats in Olds' poem more dire than the threat of exclusion, in Morrison's novel danger lurks on all sides: the baby might drown in its mother's blood or in the river water, the dirty river water might infect Sethe or her child with a fatal case of puerperal fever, the whereabouts of the runaway Sethe might be disclosed by an opportunistic Amy. (And unlike Huckleberry Finn, Sethe cannot even indulge in the act of lying down and dying, for to do so would be to consign her fetus to burial alive.) Miraculously, both Sethe and her baby defy the odds and manage to survive.

Still, for all Sethe's lack of reliance upon a divine authority, Amy invokes God, Baby Suggs addresses and knows God, and Morrison's narrator assesses what Sethe and Amy have done in words that recall the simplicity, calm, and grandeur of the Bible. After Sethe's baby is born, Morrison's narrative shifts into a sweeping panoramic scan of the landscape and a biblical appraisal of the two women's work: "On a riverbank in the cool of a summer evening two women struggled under a shower of silvery blue. They never expected to see each other again in this world and at the moment couldn't care less. But there on a summer night surrounded by bluefern they did something together appropriately and well" (84). She makes a point of how the average spectator probably would not have appreciated the magnitude and difficulty of the task at hand, accentuating the dramatic irony in the discrepancy between this imaginary viewer's dismissal of the two women as "two throw-away people, two lawless outlaws" and their actual status as courageous, capable, even heroic accomplishers of the task at hand (84). The implication is that even though Sethe does not pray to God, there is a God who bears witness to and approves of the unselfish act that these women have carried out. Morrison implies that it is not just her but God as well who approves this act as good, righteous, holy if not heroic.

Morrison's rewriting of *Huck Finn* alters the original story in several important ways, as I have noted. First of all, it is a black woman who is the protagonist and with whom we are made to identify; Sethe is no mere contrivance of the plot or idealized figure, like Jim. The white woman Amy is hardly Sethe's superior, in any way, for she makes numerous faulty assumptions about Sethe, and she is as marginal a figure as Sethe—looking malnourished, without connections, uneducated, and even a bit daft. There is something comic about Amy's quest for carmine velvet in Boston—the expensiveness of the cloth suggesting Amy's yearning for bourgeois respectability while its texture and color reflect a kind of endometrial softness, as if Amy were yearning for a nourishing bed of blood within which she could be reborn and nourished. Morrison suggests that Sethe's maternity is deeply attractive to Amy because she is starved not just for food but for the kind of emotional nurturing she imagines a post-parturient Sethe might offer. Yet Morrison resists developing this bond of the moment into any kind of sustained friendship or idealizing of either of her two characters. Amy is not a kindly abolitionist but a scrawny, uneducated bigot on an improbable quest for red velvet, and Sethe is in such desperate straits that she wants to die.

Morrison takes care not to falsify through idealization the relationship between the two women either: this is not the beginning of a beautiful friendship but a short-lived, fleeting, serendipitous encounter, and Amy almost abandons Sethe to her fate, only grudgingly returning to minister to her. Amy's speech is crude, judgmental, and not designed to comfort: "Don't up and die on me in the night, you hear?" she tells Sethe, "I don't want to see your ugly black face hankering over me" (82). Fortunately, her actions upstage and bely her unsympathetic speech; she does what needs to be done, and so manages to help preserve Sethe and her child. Some may feel that Amy is a token benevolent white character in the novel—a sop thrown to white readers—but I interpret her and the entire scene with her as an attempt on Morrison's part to re-imagine the relationship between Huck and Jim in such a way that both characters are represented unsentimentally and with respect. Racial and socioeconomic tensions of the late nineteenth century seem far more plausibly represented in Morrison's account of her interracial dyad than in Twain's, where Jim's resentment is so conspicuously absent.

Morrison slyly suggests that if Huck and Jim are afforded the luxury of escape (from the authorities, from civilization, from the cultural codes that seek to estrange them), there is no escape available for the hugely swollen Sethe: she is captive to her body and must give birth when and where that body goes into labor with the help of whomever strolls by. If Huck and Jim are forced to try to elude the authorities as they make their escape on the river, Sethe and Amy end up doing something far more difficult and far more noble. Sethe wants to die, but makes an effort at living so as not to entomb her infant. Amy could have betrayed Sethe by notifying the authorities of her whereabouts and thereby earning the reward money, but she identifies with her as a suffering being instead and passes up this opportunity. When Sethe names the child Denver, Morrison makes clear that Sethe does this not so much out of gratitude to Amy but because she likes the name; still, the effect of this naming is to confer upon Amy some small measure of unsought immortality. Just as Olds' persona insists that symbolic immortality be granted to the heroic birthers of children, so does Sethe grant a kind of symbolic immortality to her unlikely savior, a young girl who has only begun menstruating. Both Olds and Morrison recognize that value is conferred by those who have the power of naming others.

In "The Language of the Brag" (1980) and *Beloved* (1987), both Olds and Morrison represent in heroic, exalted terms those women who give birth—while using the opportunity to chide their specific male literary forefathers. Olds' persona both mocks and mimics the proud tone of Homeric warriors and those who pay tribute to their deeds, suggesting the ridiculousness of this posturing even as she adopts it for herself. Morrison is less overt in her subversions, dramatizing in *Beloved* her ideas set forth in *Playing in the Dark* that the ending of *Huckleberry Finn* does a disservice to Twain's readers by objectifying Jim, treating him not like a moral human being with feelings and a sense of indignation but as a means towards the greater end of humanizing Huck. Morrison's more plausible representation of the temporary alliance between Sethe and Amy gracefully and unobtrusively steers clear of Twain's nineteenth-century sentimentalizations and falsifications. Morrison suggests in both her critical work and her novel that there are ways to depict alliance between members of different races without objectifying either of those members. If Olds noisily and self-consciously one-ups Whitman and Ginsberg by flaunting her powers of pro/creativity, Morrison more quietly one-ups Twain, implying that women like Sethe and Amy are the greater heroes than Huck and Jim, for men can easily escape from the excesses of their sexual fortunes, but women cannot escape from their bodies. They are held captive to them throughout the process of reproduction, and there is nothing more vulnerable than a runaway slave about to give birth in the wilderness.

Notes

1. Think of Joyce's playfully perverse representation of Leopold Bloom —a little cuckold of a man who clearly relishes rather than transcends his body, insofar as he loves to eat and engage in masturbatory fantasies—as a modern day Odysseus. Woolf's Septimus Smith, Faulkner's Quentin Compson, Miller's Willie Loman—the high percentage of suicidal failures and the theme of the anti-heroic in modernist and post-modernist literature has been long noted. For writers like Olds and Morrison, then, the move from the masculine anti-heroic to the privileging of a new feminine heroine is not a terribly vast leap to make.

2. In terms of pain suffered during delivery, ether was not introduced as the first anesthetic agent until 1847 when it was used on Fanny Appleton Longfellow (Leavitt 265). The obstetrical use of chloroform was not discovered until 1831; twilight sleep was not introduced until 1914 (Leavitt 267). Moreover, the mere fact these forms of anesthesia had been discovered does not mean they were used or widely available. Debates about the merits of anesthesia raged on both scientific and religious grounds.

3. Weinstein concludes that:

Morrison understands . . . that the most artful sorts of survival start on the other side of innocence . . . The culture she brings to life in her pages has had to find the terms of its survival—and its dignity—outside the syndrome of the proper, propriety, and property. Seasoned by centuries of slavery, it has absorbed too much white abuse to envisage its own will as immaculately intact. Flexibility and a contingent, redefinable identity tend to replace Compson paralysis, Sutpen monumentality. She has no interest in mourning the collapse of a system of inheritances that never acknowledged her people in the first place . . . (192-93)

4. Jan Furman draws attention to Morrison's awareness of the freedom/enslavement dichotomy at the heart of *Huckleberry Finn:*

In reviewing the much-discussed final chapters of *Huckleberry Finn,* Morrison declares Jim's failed bid for freedom, his (re)enslavement, to be a perfect complement to Huck's liberty. The latter cannot be comprehended without the former . . . The ending is "the elaborate deferment of a necessary and necessarily unfree Africanist character's escape because freedom has no meaning to Huck or to the text without the specter of enslavement, the anodyne to individualism; the yardstick of absolute power over the life of another; the signed, marked, informing, and mutating presence of a black slave." (10)

Works Cited

Chester, Laura, ed. *Cradle and All: Women Writers on Pregnancy and Birth.* Boston: Faber and Faber, 1989.

Cosslett, Tess. *Women Writing Childbirth: Modern Discourses of Motherhood.* New York: Manchester UP, 1994.

Doyle, Laura. *Bordering on the Body: The Racial Matrix of Modern Fiction and Culture.* New York: Oxford UP, 1994.

Furman, Jan. *Toni Morrison's Fiction.* Columbia, SC: U of South Carolina P, 1996.

Homans, Margaret. *Bearing the Word: Language and Female Experience in Nineteenth-Century Women's Writing.* Chicago: U of Chicago P, 1986.

Leavitt, Judith Walzer. *Brought to Bed: Child-bearing in America, 1750-1950.* Oxford: Oxford UP, 1986.

Lester, Julius. "Morality and *Adventures of Huckleberry Finn.*" *Adventures of Huckleberry Finn: A Case Study in Critical Controversy.* Ed. Gerald Graff and James Phelan. Boston: Bedford, 1995.

Morrison, Toni. *Beloved.* New York: Plume, 1987.

——. *Playing in the Dark: Whiteness and the Literary Imagination.* Cambridge: Harvard UP, 1992.

New Shorter Oxford English Dictionary. Oxford: Oxford UP, 1993.

Olds, Sharon. *Satan Says.* Pittsburgh: Pittsburgh UP, 1980.

Rimmon-Kenan, Shlomith. "Narration, Doubt, Retrieval: Toni Morrison's Beloved." *Narrative* 4.2 (May 1996): 109-23.

Shaw, Stephanie J. "Mothering Under Slavery in the Antebellum South." *Mothering: Ideology, Experience and Agency.* Ed. Evelyn Nakano Glenn, Grace Chung, and Linda Rennie Forcey. New York: Routledge, 1994.

Weinstein, Philip M. *What Else But Love? The Ordeal of Race in Faulkner and Morrison.* New York: Columbia UP, 1996.

Wyatt, Jean. "Giving Body to the Word: The Maternal Symbolic in Toni Morrison's Beloved." *PMLA* 108 (1993): 474-88.

10

THE BIRTH OF NEW LANGUAGES

Kimberly M. Blaeser

Burlington, Wisconsin. January 29, 1996. My son is born at 8:55 p.m. In my ecstasy all language falls away. I "ooh" and "hmm" and "wow," gently trace the shape of his face as I soothe his newborn cry, touch his small clenched fists, feel the roundness of his form in my hands and snuggled against my side. His daddy and I watch as he is footprinted, washed, weighed, and measured. His emergence has enveloped us in this stillpoint. We sustain it with our silence, holding hands tightly, reading the messages in one another's eyes. After hospital ministrations, "Baby Wardzala" is returned to us. He nurses until his tiny mouth falls off my breast in sleep.

Midnight. Twenty-four hours have passed since my water broke announcing the onset of labor. Twenty-four hours of chicken broth, juices and jello. Of equal parts, ravenous, exhilarated, and exhausted, I enjoy a much too modest box lunch, relay each baby detail to my parents by phone, and manage a short nap.

2:30 a.m. With a windchill of 20 degrees below zero outside, the cold seeps in around the edges of the darkened hospital window when my hungry baby is brought to me again. Yet this bundle of newness seems to glow with warmth. The mark of a holier realm still swaddles him, glistens from his blue eyes. As I hold him against me to nurse for the second time, I feel my age falling away, my old failings vanishing in the light of his aura.

January 30, 3:30 a.m. He sleeps again. Inspired, I begin my first writing as a mother.

January 30, 4:30 p.m. Our baby's visitors wonder about a name. We consult together—again. During my pregnancy, I have campaigned for Gavin, White Hawk; his daddy for continuing the Leonard tradition from grandfather to father to son. I simply cannot hear myself using "Big Leonard" and "Little Leonard," or worse still, "Junior." Just before the records office closes we call in our decision for his birth certificate: Leonard Anthony Wardzala, named after his paternal grandfather, Leonard, and his maternal grandfather, Anthony. We will call him *Anthony*.

January 31, 8:30 a.m. Lenny is back and breathless with his news. "We have to change the baby's name." After all the effort of compromise, I am hesitant. Then he tells me. He, who never remembers his dreams, who has remained skeptical of night wisdom, has had a dream that startled him awake knowing the name was wrong. What does he want to call the baby? *"Gavin."*

February 1, 5:00 a.m. Just over two days after his birth, in the wee hours of the morning, I finish a draft of my welcome poem for Gavin Leonard Wardzala:

> motherbirth
>
> small scuttled breaths
> warm about my neck
> squeaks
> whimpers
> sighs
> tiny newborn cries
> in my dreams
> that waken
> here in half-dark room
>
> rabbit light
> falls across your bed
> between your sleep
> and mine
> between my old worn life
> and this new dream
> I stand
> half afraid
> of both
>
> canal of indecision
> floating
> as if to choose
>
> but you cry out
> here
> in this one place
> and I with you

bound now
swaddled
moving to your rhythms

swaying, rocking
cooing womb song
I hear my voice
intone heartbeats
soothing each
waking
changing
feeding
sleeping

light slides round
our days
time breathes
baby breath
slowly in and out

so new
the sound of you
but sure
as your hunger
cries red faced
from flannel wrapped wings
eyes glistening
tiny wide mouth
pulling me in
holding me
suckling
grounding me
force beyond gravity
old as time
but fresh again

Gavin
tiny White Hawk
winter night and I
welcome you

February 1, 12:00 Noon. We are driving Gavin home from the hospital when Lenny stops the car to make certain I have seen. A White Hawk swoops over us. Once, twice, and slowly, smoothly away. We celebrate the message: *Yes, we have the name right.*

First Days. Calls, notes and gifts pour in. Visitors come to greet Gavin, not the least of which includes a mid-afternoon coyote and a small herd of deer. Philip Red Eagle telephones from Washington State. "You're not going to believe this," he says, "but I saw a white hawk on the day your baby was born. We call it a swamp hawk out here." I believe it.

February 12. Lenny drives my mom and dad to the airport early this morning. It is my first day on my own caring for the baby. Of course, reassurance comes. As I walk downstairs carrying Gavin, suddenly I feel something strange and glance up. Outside the alcove window, perched on the deck rail, a huge hawk peers in at us. A moment for recognition, I voice an invitation to Gavin to look, too, and that soon the huge wings launch it away. Grateful and breathless, I watch the guardian swoop back onto the property, recede from my vision. And I stand, again searching the purity of this child's small face.

October 4, 1998. This fall I began to reflect on childbirth, motherhood and the writing life. On how we must live poetry to write it. But also on how we must nurture it as we do children, with time and attention. And who am I in this new transformation, a poetmother or a motherpoet?

"And I with you\bound now\swaddled\moving to your rhythms . . ." How much had already changed when I wrote those words—changed in me and in the patterns of my living—I little knew. I became an apprentice to the new master language of babyhood, a sometimes unwilling explorer in a chaotic dimension of parenthood. Veiled from me then in those first days of mothering was the compulsory and permanent nature of the alterations in my life.

After Gavin was born, he did not immediately begin to inhabit my dreams. When I slept I still lived my former life. A young writer on the reading circuit, late night cafe au laits, sleeping with books and scribbled lines of poems. So his cries would startle me not only awake but into another realm of experience. The duality lasted only a few nights, but I remember feeling moved and oddly stunned when I came awake one early morning knowing the old metaphysics had evaporated on a hawk's wingbeat.

My writing life, too, as I had practiced it is gone. With motherhood, both my schedule and my perspective are irretrievably altered. Writing time has become only snatched moments. Yet I write with an expanded vocabulary, a wider range of metaphor.

Boundary Waters Canoe Area Wilderness, June 20, 1996. First Day of Summer. This evening when we took the baby for his first canoe ride, a golden eagle flew over and we could hear the wings down thrust and fan the air. Hough, hough, hough. They echoed for me the sounds I made when giving birth, the blowing breaths of delivery.

Linking the music of those two moments, resulted, like fusion, in a new power, an understanding of the artistic light that pregnancy, birthing, and motherhood wrought. If a certain leisure for lingering over language had disappeared, it was replaced with a larger vision. A new poetry had awakened in me.

What is poetry if not awareness? With responsibility for a new life, I began to re-examine everything. And I had the time. Breastfeeding means sitting still. Approximately one hour out of every four I sat quietly, no distractions except my suckling child. Luckily hormones or instinct filled me with a fascination for every movement or expression that crossed that newborn face.

Still this endless immobility contrasted sharply with my former busyness. Two or three weeks of serenity was about my limit. I had become used to grading student papers and eating simultaneously, walking and writing, driving and making lists, reading while doing almost any other thing. Ten days before the baby was born, I was wallpapering. Except for sleep, I was seldom still. Suddenly I needed to stop the dash and clamor, take my focus off accomplishment.

Replace it with . . . what? Repetitive routine? "Waking, changing, feeding, sleeping?" Yes, yes, yes, and yes. But in the midst of administering that constant care, a new seeing came into my life. Finding that altered center of consciousness or accepting it, understanding it as a gift for creativity, took some time. The euphoria is there at birth and in bonding, but then comes, I admit it, boredom. Recording wet and messy diapers to keep track of intake and output, congratulating each burp, washing and sterilizing everything provides only so much stimulation and satisfaction.

Madonna, mother, matron, is that the progression? Happily not. Just when the schedules and cooing tranquillity had worn thin, I broke through to a different level of attentiveness. Perhaps this is what Zen calls mindfulness. I don't know how to characterize this perceptiveness, but it leads to moments of pure poetry, of enlightenment. One day laying with Gavin on the king-size bed upstairs, late afternoon sun blinking on and off our bodies, I suddenly recognize the perfect acorn shape of his head. His solid chin, sweet molded face, topped with the copper curves of hair. He looks and feels to me then the replica of a finely shaped acorn. A lover of acorns as Frost had been of birches, I can have no finer vision then to see in my child's face the memory of that flawless contour and color, the ripeness of fall, a delicate yet solid beauty.

At about this time I began to write short haiku-like poems, trying to capture moments like these, when time dissolves in an ecstasy of stimulation from the senses, in a flood of intuition.

> huffs of your sleeping
> breath a tiny bellows
> blowing cool across my arm

Sometimes, the poem records only the sensation. Other times, it implies the treasure of the instant, the insight or realization of connection, the channel it opens into a startling alive moment.

> plum-sized fists and berry toes
> each of your fingers and mine
> into the choir-boy O
> sweet hollow of your mouth.

> velvet tongue traces
> discovering shapes
> memorizing each
> and wetting them with life.

Motherhood like poetry consists to a large degree of letting go, relinquishing restraint and a certain kind of decorum. You are after all endlessly baring swollen breasts, swabbing the site of the severed umbilical cord, and constantly wiping mushy poop. Your focus shifts from the aesthetic to the practical. No longer was it my priority to appearing charming, coy, or cultured, well-groomed, well-educated, and well-read. Competence became the new measure. Adequate on the tired days. If I managed a shower before noon, I was doing well.

February 25, 1996. Today, for the first time since the baby was born, I wear a dress and Lenny and I take Gavin out with my family. I feel proud and especially put-together. Then I notice my walking sounds funny. I look down to discover I have two unmatched shoes on. At least they are close in color!

But beyond this shift in focus, with motherhood you cross some barrier that lets you address such things as biology and sensuality with greater honesty and humor. You give assent to experience, every kind of experience. One of my playful and graphic poems from this era catalogues the varied shapes and textures of animal droppings, pauses to "read" their messages, and pronounces: "my dog and I/devoted students of scat."

If I abandoned a bit of delicacy as I grew into motherhood, I replaced it in certain circumstances with the classic lioness ferocity. This means my child's needs supersede the frivolous desires of those around me. I have temporarily lost the willingness or patience to "mother" my adult family members, students, friends, and especially, total strangers. My husband is stunned when I "bodyblock" State Fair-goers who are about to step into Gavin's view of the horse parade. He watches in disbelief as I authoritatively instruct a souped-up car of teen-agers to relinquish a parking spot they have taken in our stead. These feats have their counterparts in poetry. I bring to my writers' group "Lament," a poem "for all the wild young girls/. . . who become their mother's clone":

> for all the giddy-
> up girls
> standing in midnight dew
> at country kegs
> and blowing their youth
> out their nostrils
>
> . . . for all tired women
> wearing life
> like some virus they caught
> whose incubation
> was twenty years.

And one of the members laughs about the unmotherly new reach and power in my voice.

Perhaps the most pervasive development of my poetic voice involves an expanded sense of history, personal and cultural. My most mundane gestures, the slight rise in my lids and eyebrows that hold Gavin's attention in supermarket lines mirrors the silent messages exchanged years on end with my own mother and hers with her mother. The recited "I'm the boss around here" as baby fists first find and pound the table speak themselves in my father's intonations, mimic the game he played with my brother and recall the stories he told of it. Baby moments continually superimpose themselves on old stories, pictures, voices, relationships.

July 17, 1996. Although I have sewn nothing but torn seams for years, tonight I finish a ribbon shirt for Gavin. The stitches joined pieces of memory as well as cloth as I recall my uncle Bill's fingers cutting and turning tobacco cans to make jingles for my dance dress, my mother patiently drawing a pattern, cutting, basting, fitting, sewing, and fasten-

ing ribbons. And I pictured my hand just last April posed flat against a pendleton blanket with Gavin's, small and dimpled, resting next to mine, each of our wrists adorned in turquoise bracelets. Gavin's first Indian jewelry from his uncle, Robert. His first Indian regalia, patterned, cut, and sewn by his mother. The patterns repeating, sweetly, sadly.

Living an awareness of imitation and continuance breeds a certain quality in poetry. A dappled light: brilliant expansion across time and distance coupled with shadows passing in melancholy. My mother's long and continuing battle with metastasized breast cancer heightened the urgency with which I gathered and stored moments, traced and shared with her the loops of our mothering, tightly secured in language the threads of history. In one long and leisurely poem I recall the "Kitchen Voices" I heard "in the crowded rooms of childhood." I then literally and symbolically transport Gavin to "my childhood's bedroom" where our dreams merge "in one hollow/of the age-worn mattress" and we listen together to the "old voices" which "ferry me across time on their currents." But even as I long for those voices to "speak on and on," to save me from the loss of meaning I fear will come with their silence, I realize my own role as the mother speaker:

> certain I am the voice of his slumber
> knowing truly it is my cadence and range
> that sings to this child a known world.

I suddenly see myself and my writing becoming reformed into a conduit of survivance. I eventually turn from my memories and even my attachment to and dependence upon those memories to the responsibility of my own voice, knowing even as I do, that my song is:

> but a simple translation
> of those ageless kitchen voices
> chanting lives
> chanting from the far side of the soul
> *sha sha sha sha*
> and *follow me.*

The duties of motherhood and poetry suddenly merge, and both expand in their insistence on the telling, the honest tracing of:

> buried vein patterns
> born of blood and devotion
> from the bed hollow of sound and history.

My poetry has always carried an awareness of Anishinaabe story, culture, and community. I consciously work to give voice to the silences of the unrepresented past of my family and my people. Now, however, I also begin to understand in a concrete way the "seventh generation" prophecies, the oratorical and instructive gestures of Indian people toward the future. The history must be carried beyond me. I am no longer "the future generation." I am the past, a small part of the present, and an even smaller part of the future.

Stawart, Michigan. July 20, 1996. Ribbon-shirted and rosy-cheeked from the morning's damp coolness, Gavin arrives for his naming ceremony. After hearing one song he joins his cooing voice to the singing and drumming. The rituals call me back. Smokey passage to clean heart. Tobacco offering. Color strips of spirit.

The language reprimands and invites me. Gavin has a place in this lodge because somewhere old ones dedicated themselves to its keeping, because our relatives spent and continue to spend pieces of their lives for community.

Learning and keeping alive the Anishinaabe language becomes more than personal. Defending the culture. Remembering the stories. These acts build the bridge from my generation to the next—to Gavin's. And if I build well, a tiny blue-eyed Indian may someday extend his memory back beyond his mother and his vision forward beyond himself. And so my writing takes up the cause anew. My poems carry the language, work to understand the pathways of tradition, repeat instructions for survival. "Recite the Names of All the Suicided Indians" recalls the high mortality rates among Indian youth:

> Obituaries
> read like tribal rolls
> he says,
> and saves his rice money.
> Memorial wreathes
> cost more each year.
> Too many die
> from lack of the language.
> Too many too young
> too Indian or too little.

With more invested now, I search the antidote to this fate and instruct: "Nagah'mo./Sing." The chorus the poem intones is one of belonging, reconnection, of naming and being able to name: "keep singing your name/your life/keep singing/your name/your life."

Naming is the proper province of the poet. And so I have a means to become the conduit of survival that motherhood inspires in me. Perhaps I tutor myself in this new role by claiming the power. In my poem, "Of Landscape and Narrative," ostensibly the re-creation of various natural encounters, I link the animal instincts and migrations with those of human communities:

> place anchors
> holds generations
> evolutions of face
> and history
> spinning
> spinning on land axis

Ultimately, I acknowledge the place of the poet, my place, in this continuance:

> memories of passages
> ranging like voices
> across my inner ear
> distances
> traced in hieroglyphs
> written in swamp meadows
> stories migrating home.

The "homing" instinct motherhood awakens in my writing and life inspires me to watch more closely the daily motions and common rituals of my family; to listen more intently to each voice, each story, each wistful word; and to concentrate my energies on retaining and then "re-membering" in language and in living the beating heart of these lives. I write my relatives memories, translate the intonations of their voices, describe posture and gesture, believing each contains some tiny part of spirit I may absorb and embody. Yet among my Indian family, even in the midst my mother's passing, the tracings I take refuse the neat delicate shape of pure nostalgia. More often the life shapes and visions draw bold, colorful lines of humor. Falling in the out-house stories come in the same breath as memories of Grandpa Antell's last gift to Grandma.

And I am reminded. My models for parenting, auntie-ing and uncle-ing come from laughing, singing, crawling-on-the-floor relatives. And so the changing voice in my motherpoetry stems also, from another kind of relinquishment and augmentation. As a mother, I let go a certain stature of propriety and freely re-member my physical and verbal playfulness. I find it fiercely more important to be nurturing then proper, even if it means singing or humming an imperfect scale of lullabies and baby songs in hallways or waiting rooms, cooing and clucking my way through phone calls, making silly faces, performing with finger puppets, or waltzing about the room with my baby bundle while discussing work schedules or revisions. Or, as I remember so vividly, doing my part of the two-person proofreading of my latest academic work in my best baby voice.

Such liberation, I found, grows with the child. Here, for the first of many times, Gavin becomes the teacher as he rewards my silliness with gurgles, squirming body, and smiles. I could say what has been said—we relearn joy, imagination, curiosity from children—and it would be true. And each of these feed our writing.

But let me speak specifically about language and our sense of the literary. Repetition reigns in child rearing. Repeat the same tasks, read the same stories, sing the same songs, recite the same rhymes, list the same directions, and later, watch the same videos, over and over and over and over. Such repetition for awhile seemed to drive my dreaming self underground. I performed on rote and "lived" elsewhere. But when so much of my "real" life consisted of similar tasks, I began to learn to bring them alive. Whether through voice, mime, or other imaginative play, I interjected newness into the routines.

As a writer, this meant the birth or expansion of my creativity. Doesn't the literary canon consist of the same stories, plots and circumstances, given in variation? Aren't the moon, the love relationship, and death the same subjects poetry must always remake anew? Can child-rearing really allow me to practice at writing? Only if I let it.

In the circumstances of motherhood, I also began to relearn the comfort and value of repetition in life and writing. As someone from a Native American background, I have always been immersed in the storytelling tradition and the purposeful repetition that it often involves. Not only do individual oral performances repeat certain key phrases, but the canon of community or tribal stories weaves together in a patterned variation the retelling of whole incidents, stories, and relationships. For retention, reinforcement, re-membering, renewal. Poetry likewise explores intervals and avenues of re-speaking.

One of my poetmother experiments brought me a sounder appreciation of poetic form. I decided that the pantoum with its patterned and interlocking repetition might be the ideal form for a motherhood poem. In my experimentation, I discovered the dual motives of rekindling and expansion intended and available in such a pattern.

Baby Pantoum

Now I lay you down to sleep
Hush now, hush now my little son,
Pray you please the quiet keep
Now that this long day is done.

Hush now, hush now my little son
Diaper dry and just now fed,
Now that this long day is done
It's high time you went to bed.

Diaper dry and just now fed
You've heard each song I know in turn,
It's high time you went to bed—
Ah, there must be other lullabies to learn.

You've heard each song I know in turn
Played peek-a-boo and patty cake,
Ah, there must be other lullabies to learn.
Or some new parent class to take.

Played peek-a-boo and patty cake,
Rushed to wash and dry and fold;
Some new parent class to take,
With this little mind to mold

Rushed to wash and dry and fold
Mashed bananas, baked fresh bread,
With this little mind to mold
There's never time to rest my head.

Mashed bananas, baked fresh bread.
And wondered again did I do alright?
There's never time to rest my head.
And when will he sleep the night?

And wondered again will I do alright
Winter's ginger-haired baby child?
And will you ever sleep the night?
Sun has set and evening's mild.

Winter's ginger-haired baby child,
Pray you please the quiet keep.
Sun has set and evening's mild,
Now I lay you down to sleep.

Indeed, re-speaking and motherhood might be synonymous as might re-speaking and childhood. Isn't it the greatest joy to hear your own child's sweet (and, in Gavin's case, deep) little voice repeat first words, the words you have said over and over to him or her? How they charm us with mimicry, imitating our tones, gestures, and phrases. How they enlighten us as well. What deeper well of poetic material than a child's mirroring? And, whether delighted by sweet imitation or privately chastised by its unflinching truthfulness, we watch for and celebrate when we see ourselves, our spouses, our relatives in our child's behavior.

February 14, 1996. Tonight as my little Valentine and I fall asleep together, I suddenly recognize the slight side to side settling motion of his head as he cocoons into sleep. It has lulled me these many years. How fearful and awesome the passing of even this smallest animal ritual.

Yes, lives renew themselves in children. Through them we revive all past fascinations—perhaps the natural most of all. *Where dat ladybug live? Why do sun shine? What do giraffe-es eat?* Children notice things: colors, shapes, scents, sounds. They fearlessly leap to experience and carry us along: tasting raindrops, chasing lightning bugs, lying in soft moss, collecting everything from rocks to butterflies to pinecones. They never tire of telling the stories of the world as they see it. Gavin's first "poem" was recited from October through December just before he turned two: "Big daddy deer cross road/Mama deer stay field/Baby deer road, too." Their interpretations as well as their why, why, whys remind us of mysteries we have not yet solved, of the wonders we live, of the stuff of poetry.

Nowhere has that wonder been more rewarding for me than in the arena of language. Babble, baby song, invented words, signature intonation, mispronunciations, I've enjoyed each one as it unfolds. To say it has enriched my appreciation of language grossly understates the wealth of blessings that comes with the melodic ring of baby talk. Yet hearing my son acquire language has clearly altered my sense of sound, rhythm, and poetic relationship. I witnessed, for example, the very visual quality he brings to language, the literal way he interprets colloquial expressions, and the rapid synapses triggered by new words. When learning colors, he wanted every word—nouns, verbs and adjectives—to possess one. "What color run? Is bigger purple, mama?" But perhaps the sweetest, most endearing (and most quotable) learning pattern is the way he brings to the hearing and speaking of unfamiliar words words he already knows. When he heard his paternal grandfather pretend to ride a horse, he imitated his grandpa's command by calling out, "Kitty-up, kitty-up!"

When something becomes very wet it is "soaped." In the rural area where we live, many people drive "picnic trucks." When something is turned over it is "up-ducky-down." Poetmother that I am, I attempt to capture the inspiration of his whimsical language magic.

> Up-Ducky-Down
> You turn the world
> "Kitty-up, kitty-up!"
> with your call.
> Gleefully rocking my heart,
> your wooden neigh-neigh,
> the stodgy sense of sounds—
> go up-ducky-down.
> And memory and attachment
> rent space in our house
> count "1,2,3,4...3,4...3,4."
> Identities, Imeyou
> swittling together.
> "Mama carry you!"
> While big grrr, little grrr
> and tigrr
> keep changing their clothes
> kissing their reflections
> "he backwards"
> and clapping their hands.
> Ambition goes up-ducky-down
> "Now you turn go kitty-up"
> and I do.

At times ambition may graciously step aside for motherhood. At other times, it pounds loudly at my temples while I am bathing the baby or trying to fall back to sleep after a night waking. As a mother, I jealously guard my time with Gavin. As a writer, I lament the loss of my own time, the tired slow progression of my work, my falling out of the writing/publishing/speaking/reading "network." The year I was pregnant with Gavin, I traveled to twenty-six different locations to give readings and speak at conferences. This past year, perhaps twelve. My publications continue to trickle out, but I miss twice as many opportunities to submit as I can take advantage of. Still when I shut myself away for an evening to write or travel to do a reading, I long to be with him, fear I might miss some special moment, worry he will be lonely, get hurt, be somehow harmed by my absence. If I hear his little voice wail or see his sweet acorn face pressed against the glass of my library door at home, I will usually put away my writing and open my door to the new and fleeting poetry of motherhood.

October 6, 1998. Gavin runs to me with photos he has found and wants to look at together. They are a mixture, some taken before his birth, some more recently. We look at a photograph of him and his father in the Boundary Waters Canoe Area Wilderness. After a second of enjoyment, he asks, "Where's Mama?" I try to explain that I am taking the picture. That doesn't satisfy. "Mama's not on the picture, but she would be right about here if you use your imagination." "Where my im-mag-in-nay-shun?" "In your mind." "Where my mind?" "In your sweet little head."

Finally we get on to other pictures. Now comes the real challenge. There is Mommy and Daddy together, no Gavin, years before Gavin came along. "Where Gavin in this picture?" But I'm a poetmother now. I've had practice. "He's in Mommy and Daddy's imagination." "In your sweet little heads?" "Yes."

Along with the next poem and the next baby, I add in my im-mag-in-nay-shun.

CONTRIBUTORS

Ellen Argyros is an Assistant Professor of English at the University of Wisconsin–Fox Valley. Her first book, *The Limits of Sympathy in George Eliot's Novels* (Peter Lang Press), is forthcoming. She is currently working on a compilation of essays on representations of maternal subjectivity in the works of George Eliot, Toni Morrison, Harriet Beecher Stowe, and Virginia Woolf. She has also published articles on Elizabeth Griffith and on teaching as a mother. She lives in Appleton with her husband and two sons.

Debra Beilke is an Assistant Professor of English at Concordia University–St. Paul, where she teaches writing, American literature and African literature. She has published articles and presented papers on writers such as Zora Neale Hurston, Ellen Glasgow, Dorothy Parker, Erskine Caldwell, William Faulkner, and Bessie Head. She is currently working on a book-length manuscript on identity and humor in Southern Renaissance fiction.

Kimberly M. Blaeser, an Associate Professor of English at the University of Wisconsin–Milwaukee, teaches courses in Creative Writing, Native American Literature, and American Nature Writing. Of Anishinaabe and German ancestry, Blaeser is an enrolled member of the Minnesota Chippewa Tribe, and grew up on the White Earth Reservation in Northwestern Minnesota. Blaeser's publications include a collection of peotry, *Trailing You,* which won the 1993 First Book Award from the Native Writers' Circle of the Americas and a critical study *Gerald Vizenor: Writing in the Oral Tradition.* Her poetry, short fiction, personal essays, and scholarly articles have been anthologized in over fifty Canadian and American collections including *Earth Song, Sky Spirit, Narrative Chance, Returning the Gift, Women on Hunting, The Colour of Resistance, New Voices in Native American Literary Criticism, Blue Dawn, Red Earth, Unsettling American, Dreaming History, Reinventing the Enemy's Language,* and *As We Are Now.* Blaeser is also the editor of a collection of Anishinaabe prose, *Stories Migrating Home,* from Loonfeather Press, and she is working on her second collection of poems, tentatively entitled *Absentee Indians.*

Brenda Daly, the mother of one child, a 35-year-old son, and Professor of English and Women's Studies at Iowa State University, is the author of many essays, most about contemporary novels by women. She has written two books, *Authoring a Life: A Woman's Survival in and through Literary Studies* (SUNY Press, 1998) and *Lavish Self-Divisions: The Novels of Joyce Carol Oates* (Mississippi, 1996). She also co-edited the collection, *Narrating Mothers: Theorizing Maternal Subjectivities* (Tennessee, 1991) with Maureen Reddy and is, at present, working on another book about contemporary American culture and its reception of incest narratives by women.

Karen Haas-Howland is an award-winning singer, poet, nurse, and mother of Chloe. She wrote a screenplay that is being considered by a major motion picture company. She received her master's in creative writing from UW–Milwaukee where she has been Poetry Editor of *Cream City Review* for three years. She enjoys performing her work to audiences near and far and has been featured on cable shows and public radio. She facilitates women's writing circles in the community and revels in the power of the spoken word.

Gail Lippincott is a doctoral candidate in Rhetoric and Technical and Scientific Communication at the University of Minnesota. Her research interests focus on audience awareness, including gender and disability issues, in historical and contemporary technical communication. She is completing her dissertation on the rhetorical strategies of Ellen Swallow Richards, a part of which is published as "Experimenting at Home: Writing for the Nineteenth-Century Domestic Workplace" in *Technical Communication Quarterly*.

Susan MacCallum-Whitcomb holds a Ph.D. in English from the University of New Brunswick and has been granted awards by the University of Toronto, the University of New Brunswick and the Social Science and Humanities Research Council of Canada. She teaches American literature at the University of New Brunswick (Saint John). Her special field is contemporary American poetry, and her current areas of research are American Women's Poetry and American Maternity Literature. She is particularly proud to have participated in both the ground-breaking session on Maternity Literature held at the 1996 Midwest MLA Annual Convention and the first international conference on Mothers and Daughters held at York University in 1997. Her most recent article, "Bitches with Broom Sticks: The Bad Mother in American Maternity Poetry" appears in *Mothers and Daughters at the New Millennium* (Rowman and Littlefield, 1999). A feminist activist and member of the advisory board for the Association for Research on Mothering, Susan lives in Saint John with her husband and two young children.

Andrea O'Reilly, Ph.D., is an Assistant Professor in the School of Women's Studies at York University where she teaches courses on Toni Morrison, on motherhood, and on mothers and daughters. She has presented her research at numerous international conferences and she is author of more than a dozen articles and chapters on this topic. She is co-editor of *Redefining Motherhood: Changing Patterns and Identities* (Second Story Press, 1998) and *Mothers and Daughters at the New Millennium* (Rowman and Littlefield, 1999). She is the author of *Toni Morrison on Motherhood* (forthcoming from Ohio State Press). She is currently editing *Mothers and Sons in Literature* and *Mothers and Sons: Feminist Perspectives*. She was co-ordinator of the first-ever international conferences on Mothers and Daughters (1997), and Mothers and Sons (1998) hosted by the Centre for Feminist Research, York University. O'Reilly is founding president of the Association for Research on Mothers (A.R.M.). In 1998 she was the recipient of the "University Wide" Teaching Award at York University. She has conducted numerous community workshops on motherhood, mothers and daughters, and mothers and sons. Andrea and her common-law spouse of sixteen years are the parents of a fourteen-year-old son and two daughters, ages nine and eleven.

Michele Lise Tarter is an Assistant Professor of English at The College of New Jersey. She has published several articles on early American women's writings and is co-editor of a collection of essays titled *"A Centre of Wonders": The Body in Early America* (Cornell University Press, 2000). She is currently completing her book manuscript on trans-Atlantic Quaker women, *The Body as Testimony: Quaker Women's Prophesyings in Early American Culture and Text*.

Julie Tharp received her Ph.D. from the University of Minnesota. She teaches English and Women's Studies at the University of Wisconsin–Marshfield/Wood County where she is an Associate Professor. She co-edited *Creating Safe Space: Violence and Women's Writing* with Tomoko Kuribayashi and has published a number of articles on writing by women of color, Louise Erdrich, Helena Maria Viramontes, and Joy Kogawa in particular. Other research interests include feminist film criticism and Native American quilting. She has given birth to a daughter and a son.